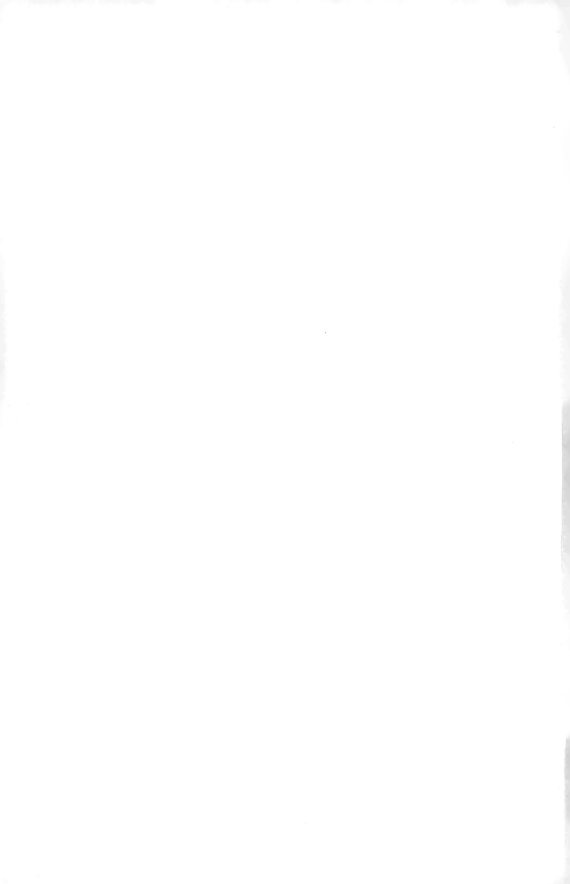

CAN MEDICINE BE CURED?

SEAMUS O'MAHONY spent many years working
for the National Health Service in Britain. He now
lives and practises medicine in his native Cork, in
the south of Ireland. His acclaimed first book, *The
Way We Die Now*, was published in 2016, and has
been translated into Swedish and Japanese.
It won a BMA Book Award in 2017.

CAN MEDICINE BE CURED?

THE CORRUPTION OF A PROFESSION

SEAMUS O'MAHONY

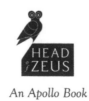

An Apollo Book

This is an Apollo Book, first published in the UK in 2019
by Head of Zeus Ltd

9 7 5   4 6 8

A catalogue record for this book is available from
the British Library.

ISBN (HB): 9781788544542
ISBN (E): 9781788544535

Typeset by Adrian McLaughlin

Printed and bound in Great Brit
CPI Group (UK) Ltd, Croydon c

Head of Zeus Ltd
First Floor East
5–8 Hardwick Street
London EC1R 4RG

WWW.HEADOFZEUS.COM

This book is dedicated to the memory of
Julia O'Connor (1924–2018)

CONTENTS

CAN MEDICINE BE CURED?

I

'PEOPLE LIVE SO LONG NOW'

We take our health for granted, a luxury unknown throughout most of human history. My mother was born in 1932, in a rural hamlet in West Cork, the youngest of nine children. When she was ten years old, she fell seriously ill. It was unusual to summon the doctor in those days, but her parents were so worried that the local GP was called. The doctor drove the ten miles from his surgery, and arrived in bad temper. He examined the child, and told her parents that she had pneumonia. He prescribed sulfapyridine, an antibacterial drug developed only a couple of years before, and known colloquially as 'M&B', after the manufacturer, May & Baker. Sulfapyridine was commonly used during the Second World War, but fell into disuse when penicillin became widely available. The GP also ordered my grandparents, for reasons which I can't fathom, on no account to give her water. They would not countenance going against the doctor's advice, and my mother endured the torments of both the pneumonia and a raging thirst. She was saved by her sister, Margaret, who under cover of night went to the well and fetched water. Whether because of her sister's forbidden ministrations, or the M&B tablets, or both, my mother survived.

Her brother Billy was not so lucky. At the age of seventeen, while at boarding school, he became ill; he had lost weight and complained of pains in his back. He was sent home, and eventually was diagnosed with spinal tuberculosis (TB). At his school – a seminary – he was in close proximity to hundreds of other boys, several of whom must have been infected with TB. The prison-like food rations (exacerbated by wartime shortages) meant that these boys were chronically malnourished, and thus more susceptible to infection. There was no effective drug treatment for TB at that time. His parents chose not to send Billy to hospital; the doctor told them that his disease was advanced and incurable, and nothing could be done for him. His mother nursed him at home; the local women rallied to her aid, looking after the house and the children. Billy died in 1946, aged eighteen. His sister, Julia, who had entered the Loreto order of nuns a few years before, was not allowed to leave the convent to attend his funeral. She died, aged ninety-four, during the writing of this book.

Tuberculosis was a blight on Ireland throughout the nineteenth century and the first half of the twentieth century.

William Wilde (father of Oscar) worked as a census commissioner, and estimated that between 1831 and 1841, TB caused 11.4 per cent (135,590 of 1,187,374) of all deaths in the country. The disease carried a social stigma, as it was associated with poverty and malnutrition, and was known by a variety of euphemisms, such as 'decline' and 'delicacy'. So great was this stigma that many sufferers were hidden away by their families. In 1948, two years after Billy's death, a young doctor called Noël Browne was appointed health minister in the new Irish coalition government. He introduced mass population screening for TB, along with BCG vaccination (Bacillus Calmette-Guérin vaccine, the standard immunization against tuberculosis). Browne's programme was moderately successful; the tuberculosis death rate dropped from 123 per 100,000 of the population in 1947 to 73 per 100,000 in 1951. He funded the construction of several new 'sanatoria' – specialist hospitals for the treatment of TB patients. Sanatoria had been well established in continental Europe since the mid-nineteenth century; Thomas Mann's *The Magic Mountain* is set in a Swiss TB clinic. The sanatoria offered bed rest, fresh air, sunshine and nutritional supplements such as cod liver oil. Some recovered under this regime; many died. A variety of surgical procedures were carried out on patients with pulmonary TB, including pneumothorax (collapsing the lung to 'rest' it), crushing of the phrenic nerve to paralyse the diaphragm (also to 'rest' the lung) and partial pneumonectomy (removal of a portion of an infected lung). These procedures were of dubious and unproven benefit. I still see elderly people who survived them.

Around the time of Billy's death, streptomycin became available for treatment of TB in the US, but it would be several years before British companies started producing the drug. In 1948, George Orwell was one of the first TB sufferers in Britain to be treated with streptomycin. Through his connections with David Astor, the editor of the *Observer*, and the health minister Aneurin Bevan, a supply of streptomycin was obtained from the US. Royalties from *Animal Farm* paid for the drug. Orwell, unfortunately, did not respond, suffering severe side effects. He donated whatever streptomycin was left over to Hairmyres Hospital near Glasgow, where he was treated. Two doctors' wives received the drug, and both were cured of their TB. The Medical Research Council started recruiting patients into their streptomycin trial in 1946. It was the first ever 'randomized controlled trial': i.e. patients were randomly allocated (to eliminate bias), in equal numbers, to the active drug (streptomycin) and a placebo, or control. The trial was concluded in 1948; it showed clearly and unambiguously that streptomycin was effective. With the advent of streptomycin, and later, other more effective drugs, deaths from TB continued to fall. Some argued that the disease was on the decline anyway, long before these drugs became available. TB hasn't gone away; it still kills millions of people in poor countries. In Ireland, the disease lingers on, targeting the poor, the marginalized, the old and immigrants. TB patients are now generally treated at home, and the sanatoria have been put to other uses. The Cork sanatorium, St Stephen's Hospital, is now a psychiatric hospital, grappling with a new blight. My mother's father was also stricken with TB (of the lungs), and spent several months in the late 1960s in St Stephen's. Children were not allowed to visit, so he would wave at us from a balcony on the first floor, a distant, ghostly, solitary figure. He was born in Lowell, Massachusetts in 1887. His father died in his early thirties of typhoid fever, forcing his widowed mother to return to Ireland and the charity of relatives. Typhoid, which once killed millions, has all but disappeared, due to vaccination and sanitation.

In 1956, there was an epidemic in Co. Cork of the viral disease poliomyelitis, or 'polio' as it is widely known. Hundreds of children contracted the disease, which causes paralysis and wasting of muscles. Some, whose chest muscles were paralysed, had to live within an 'iron lung' to survive. Many others, like the great Middle East correspondent Patrick Cockburn, endured long hospitalizations, and later, numerous orthopaedic operations. Thousands fled the city, which was effectively quarantined. The survivors of this epidemic are now in their sixties and early seventies, easily identifiable by the lifelong disability caused by polio. In the mid-1990s there were between 7,500 and 10,000 survivors of the disease still alive in Ireland. Cockburn wrote of polio in his memoir *The Broken Boy*: 'As a killer it never compared with cholera, typhus, malaria, yellow fever or consumption, but it carried an extra charge of fear because like leprosy and smallpox it disfigured and disabled the living. Aids is the only disease in the last half-century to create comparable terror.' The American virologist Jonas Salk had been working on a vaccine against polio since the early 1950s; in 1955, he announced the results of the first trial of his vaccine, which proved beyond doubt that it worked. The Salk vaccine was given by injection; it was replaced with Albert Sabin's oral vaccine in 1961. This was the vaccine I was given – taken with a lump of sugar – as a schoolboy. Polio – at least in the rich West – has disappeared.

The deaths of children and teenagers like Billy were a common tragedy for most of human history; a stroll through any old cemetery is a roll call of lost children. But something radical happened in the first half of the twentieth century. The infectious diseases which claimed the lives of so many children and young adults became curable or preventable by vaccination. Between 1885 and 1985 infant mortality in the US and Europe dropped from 140 per 1,000 (1 in 7 babies died) to 5 per 1,000 (1 in 200). Life expectancy rose from 50 to nearly 80. In 1930, maternal mortality in England was 1 in 250; it is now 8 per 100,000 (1 in 12,500). The death of a mother in childbirth is now so rare that when it does occur, it is often a national scandal. Most people with TB can be cured with prolonged antibiotic treatment. Smallpox killed more people (hundreds of millions) than the Black Death and the two world wars combined: in 1980 the World Health Organization declared it eradicated. Medicine, which for most of its history had very limited powers, was quite suddenly marvellously, miraculously effective. There was a golden age of about fifty years, from the mid-1930s to the mid-1980s, when almost anything seemed possible. Lewis Thomas (1913–93), the American doctor and essayist, wrote that when he qualified in the 1930s, 'the major threats to human life were tuberculosis, tetanus, syphilis, rheumatic fever, pneumonia, meningitis, polio, and septicaemia of all sorts. These things worried us then the way cancer, heart disease and stroke worry us today. The big problems of the 1930s and 1940s have literally vanished.'

I studied medicine from 1977 to 1983, towards the end of the golden age. Around this time, some critics began to question medicine's hegemony: the greatest of these critics was Ivan Illich. Illich (1926–2002) was an Austrian priest, philosopher and social critic. His book *Medical Nemesis* (1975) opened with the famous and, to me at the time, intoxicating assertion: 'The medical establishment has become a major threat to health.' A superstar public intellectual in the 1970s, Illich is now all but forgotten. His central theme was that institutionalization had corrupted Western civilization. Modern institutions were characterized by what Illich called 'paradoxical counterproductivity', that is, they frustrated the very purpose for which they were originally designed. Thus, formal education led to ignorance, modern transport caused gridlock and environmental despoliation, and health care was sickening. He elaborated these ideas in a series of books published between 1970 and 1975, including *Deschooling Society, Tools for Conviviality*, and – most famously – *Medical Nemesis*. This brilliant polyglot was mobbed when he appeared at universities; when he spoke at University College Dublin in 1978, 8,000 people turned up. In Edinburgh in 1974, a medical student called Richard Smith (later editor of the *British Medical Journal*) was transfixed: 'The closest I ever came to a religious experience was listening to Ivan Illich. A charismatic and passionate man surrounded by the fossils of the academic hierarchy in Edinburgh...' Illich argued that scientific medicine had little effect on the overall health of populations; this argument had been made by others, most notably the epidemiologist Thomas McKeown, who believed that sanitation, nutrition and housing were more important determinants of health. McKeown thought that doctors contributed little to health, but Illich went even further, arguing that they were actively dangerous. He attacked institutionalized modern medicine because he saw it as a new religion, with its own rituals and dogma, and the medical profession as a new priesthood. He railed against the monopoly and dominance of doctors: 'Modern medicine is a negation of health. It isn't organized to serve human health, but only itself, as an institution. It makes more people sick than it heals.'

This was heady stuff. One of Illich's many disciples was

John Bradshaw, an English doctor who had abandoned medicine for writing. His 1978 book *Doctors on Trial* was an homage to Illich and a reworking of the arguments of *Medical Nemesis*; the introduction, naturally, was written by the great man. Bradshaw often used the word 'prophet' when referring to Illich, and saw himself as the interpreter of the Austrian's more obscure pronouncements – John the Baptist to Illich's Jesus. Bradshaw was one of the speakers at my university's debating union in 1981, addressing the Illichian motion that 'Medicine has become a threat to health'. The debate was a riotous event. Several doctors spoke against the motion, which they regarded as ludicrous, and dismissed Illich and Bradshaw as cranks. I sought out Bradshaw in the college bar, and over drinks we talked animatedly about our mutual hero, Ivan Illich. Later, as I walked home, intoxicated by the debate and the beer, I wondered what I was doing, training for a profession which had 'become a threat to health'.

More than most professions, medicine colonizes one's life. After graduation, I was consumed by the demands of the job. Years went by in a blur of weekends on call and post-graduate examinations. My horizon was always near: the next job, the next qualification. For many years, I embraced this way of living and thinking. It is not without its advantages: medical career structures, and what passes for success in the profession, are so rigid and clearly laid out that the true careerist knows instinctively what to do in any given situation. I slowly ascended the ladder to the status of consultant in a

British National Health Service teaching hospital, spending many years along the way in various training positions. As a young consultant, I became something of a Pharisee, a vector of institutional and professional culture. By the age of forty, I had achieved a state of perpetual busyness, and might have continued along this well-trodden pathway for the remainder of my career. A series of events during my forties changed everything; the details are both too tedious and too personal to recount here. When, at the age of fifty, I surveyed the wreckage, I concluded that I had somehow sabotaged this promising career. The sabotage may have been subconsciously deliberate: the real problem was a loss of faith, an apostasy. The cartoon character Wile E. Coyote falls to his doom in the canyon only when he no longer *believes*; as long as he is unaware of his situation, he remains blissfully suspended in mid-air. My apostasy did not extend to the clinical encounter, and old-fashioned doctoring. I lost faith in all the other things: medical research, managerialism, protocols, metrics, even progress. I became convinced that medicine had become an industrialized culture of excess, and that Ivan Illich's assertion that it had become a threat to health – which seemed ludicrous to many doctors in the mid-1970s – was true.

I qualified just as the golden age of medicine was ending. In the thirty-five years since then, I have worked in three countries and many hospitals. I have witnessed the public's disenchantment with medicine, the emergence and global domination of what might be called the medical–industrial complex, and the corruption of my profession. This medical–industrial complex includes not just the traditional villain known as Big Pharma, but many other professional and commercial groups, including biomedical research, the health-food industries, medical devices manufacturers, professional bodies such as the royal colleges, medical schools, insurance companies, health charities, the ever-increasing regulatory and audit sector, and secondary parasitic professions such as lobbyists and management consultants.

Every age has its own foolishness, and medicine is a great barometer of contemporary fads, an 'early adopter' of new technologies and new fashions in personal behaviour, management and education. Far from being conservative and resistant to change, the medical profession forms new enthusiasms with alarming haste. If you want to know what will exercise the world next year, look at what medicine is excited about now. Doctors, both researchers and clinicians, have adopted the language, ethos and mindset of marketing: We're All in Sales Now.

Medicine has extended its dominion over nearly every aspect of human life. In doing so, it raised expectations such that disappointment was inevitable. My professional lifetime started at the end of the golden age and the beginning of the age of unmet and unrealistic expectations, the age of disappointment. Patients, doctors and society at large are the victims, dupes and slaves of this medical–industrial complex.

We are treating, and over-treating, but not healing. After three-and-a-half decades, I look back with a mixture of amusement, perplexity and shame.

I asked my mother about her bout of pneumonia and the death of her brother. Billy's death, she said, was a tragedy from which her parents never recovered. As I write, Ireland is in the throes of a medico-political crisis, because screening for cervical cancer by smear testing failed to detect pre-cancerous changes in some women. Although this type of screening has a recognized false negative, or 'miss', rate, the media and some opportunist politicians have created an atmosphere of popular outrage. 'People say how bad the health service is now,' my mother mused, 'but they should go back to the 1940s and they would see what bad care was really like. All the problems we have are because people live so long now.'

2

THE GREATEST BREAKTHROUGH
SINCE LUNCHTIME

Since the 1980s, medical research has become a global business and driver of economies; it is the intellectual motor of the medical–industrial complex. It is seen by the general public as a worthy philanthropic endeavour, carried out by altruists motivated only by a thirst for truth and a passion to cure disease and save lives. Many charities collect money to fund this noble activity, and these bodies have themselves become a substantial business sector. There is a broad societal consensus that medical research is a good thing, and the more money spent on it the better. The many people who give money to these charities might be surprised to learn that the great majority of medical research is a waste of time and money. There are two reasons for this waste: first, the vast majority of it is badly carried out, and second, research serves mainly the needs of the researchers and allied commercial interests.

My experience of working for nearly three years as a research fellow taught me quite a lot about this strange sub-culture. Research fellows are junior doctors – usually with a few years of clinical experience – who step out of clinical employment for a period to work towards a doctoral-level degree, such as an MD or a PhD. My reason for doing it was the same as nearly all other doctors: career advancement. Hospital medicine in the 1980s was highly competitive. Consultant posts generally only became available because of retirement or death and many jobs attracted twenty or more highly qualified applicants. The training posts, such as registrar and senior registrar, were nearly as competitive, and the academic portion of one's CV assumed great impor-tance. Candidates were often judged more on their research record than their clinical skills. Ambitious trainee doctors were thus heavily incentivized to publish papers in the medical journals and to obtain doctoral degrees. After three years of house officer jobs at my local teaching hospital, I had drifted into a job as registrar in gastroenterology. This choice was dictated mainly by chance and expediency; I had no burning desire to pursue a career in this speciality, over, say, one in cardiology. It was simply the job I was offered. If I was to progress in this speciality, I would have to leave Ireland, as specialist training there was almost non-existent in the 1980s. I discussed the matter with one of the local consultants, who suggested that I try my luck in Edinburgh, for no better reason than he had himself trained there. He wrote on my behalf to the professor of gastroenterology, and I went over to meet him. I was offered a job on the spot as a research fellow, which would be funded by a drug company. At that time, the pharmaceutical industry spent a lot of money on such posts, particularly in gastroenterology. This financial support purchased goodwill with the medical academics, and was tax efficient. The professor explained that I would be required to do a small trial for this drug company, but that this work would occupy only a little of my time. The main focus of my research would be the immune system of the gut.

When I started this post, I met the professor, expecting clear directions for my research. His advice, however, was vague: he suggested that I spend a few weeks in the library 'reading the literature' and learn some basic laboratory techniques. In the hospital library, I pored over papers on the intestinal immune system, a subject of indescribable dullness. I shared a laboratory bench with two shy Italians, who showed me how to 'microdissect' a biopsy from the small intestine, and stain it with various dyes, so that cell types could be counted. This counting was done by peering down a microscope at an intestinal biopsy, and clicking a manual counter every time a particular cell-type was seen. I spent many hours and days counting populations of a cell called the intra-epithelial lymphocyte. Although a helpful technician showed me the basic technique of measuring anti-body levels, I soon learned that the laboratory staff resented the research fellows, quite correctly regarding them as careerist dilettantes. My professor was proud that his many research fellows came from all over the world, and the lab coffee room displayed a map of the world with a little flag on the country of origin of each lucky pilgrim.

The study which paid my wages was a trial of a new drug for coeliac disease. It had been known since the late 1940s that coeliac disease can be treated very effectively by removing gluten from the diet. Why a drug should be mooted as a treatment for this disease is astonishing, but the idea is still seriously advocated, on the rather spurious grounds that some patients find the diet difficult to adhere to. The trial had been started by one of the Italians; I took it over, recruiting more patients. The patients had a pre-trial small intestinal biopsy, were told to continue on a normal diet, took this drug for three months, and then had another biopsy to see if there was any improvement. (The improvement with diet in coeliac disease can be seen in small intestinal biopsies.) The trial was ethically suspect, as there was no plausible biological basis why this drug, or indeed any drug, should be used as a treatment for a condition which already had a known dietary cause, and a known 'cure'. Not surprisingly, the trial showed no benefit from this drug. One patient died shortly after the conclusion of the trial, of a rare intestinal cancer associated with coeliac disease. I do not think the drug was directly to blame, but the fact that she was advised to continue eating gluten for the duration of the trial while she took this ineffective agent surely did not help. I was of course keen to publish a paper on the trial, but we were contractually obliged by the drug company to show them any such paper before submission to a medical journal. Naturally, they were against publishing the findings, as it showed no benefit from their product. They needn't have worried – the journal I sent it to rejected the paper without even sending it out for review. This was my first experience of the phenomenon of 'negative publication bias', i.e. rejection of papers describing trials with a 'negative' result.

When I tried to get my professor to point me in the direction of a specific research project, he suggested that I should develop a technique of counting cells in intestinal biopsies automatically, using a computerized system called image analysis. We never discussed anything as scientifically hifalutin as a hypothesis, a question: the main concern was to develop a new technique to generate data. He arranged for me and a lab technician called Jim to work on this at another department at the university. Jim and I spent many fruitless hours on this image analysis, but the only images we could conjure looked like interference on a television set. After several frustrating weeks, we concluded that we couldn't get any useful information using this technology. I reported back to my boss the lack of progress with the image analysis. The only option was to start again, with a new project. My professor had made his name in the 1970s with research conducted mainly on mice, and he had decided to shift the focus of his attention to humans. He was keen on adapting an animal technique called 'whole gut lavage' to humans, and I was given the task of developing this. I paid volunteers to drink four litres of an isotonic fluid called GoLytely, a laxative used to prepare patients for colonoscopy. When the volunteers were shitting clear, lager-coloured fluid, I collected this effluent, strained and filtered it, and added various chemicals to preserve the antibodies in this 'lavage fluid'. I spent hours hanging around hospital toilets, peering into steel bedpans full of faecal fluid to see if it was ready for filtering. You can get used to anything. My paid volunteers were usually Dougie and Ewan, the foul-mouthed technicians from the animal unit, who were always short of cash. A cynical contemporary of mine once defined a mouse as 'an animal which if killed in sufficient numbers produces a PhD'; the Animal Unit housed all of these poor mice, as well as monkeys and – it was rumoured – goats. I managed to avoid killing any of these innocent animals, but I was taken one morning to the Animal Unit by one of the Italians, who expertly dispatched a mouse with a flick of his wrist, swinging it by the tail and smashing its head on the edge of the laboratory counter.

The old cliché about all the world looking like a nail to a man with a hammer sums up much of medical research, and certainly mine. I was soon subjecting real patients to 'whole gut lavage' – most were preparing for colonoscopy anyway, but some weren't. I used this gut lavage technique to measure antibodies to all sorts of things, and published on them all. I applied the technique (if you can call it a technique) to everything I could think of from Crohn's disease to a type of arthritis called ankylosing spondylitis. Another more fastidious research fellow collected saliva – much less offensive to the eye and nose than my work – and he, too, looked at every possible comparison and combination of salivary antibodies. Instead of starting with a question, or a hypothesis, we began with a technique, and then produced as many data as possible. I spent two years collecting 'whole gut lavage fluid', intestinal juice, saliva and blood from various groups of patients and diseases. Over the next two years, I published several papers and wrote up my doctoral thesis. Flushed with this modest success, I foolishly formed the notion that I would make a career in research and was appointed to a more senior post in the same unit. This was a mistake, and I soon became disenchanted with academic life. After less than eighteen months in this post, I left to take up a job as senior registrar in Yorkshire. My research career, which petered out ignominiously, did, however, give me some very hard-won insight. I realized that I lacked the curiosity of the true scientist. I could have advanced as a medical academic by the conventional route, but had a low tolerance for boredom and, although cynical, I was not quite cynical enough. I was proud to have my paper in the *Lancet* and my MD degree, but that was enough, and I was relieved to move back into clinical work. The three years I spent as a research fellow were well spent from a purely utilitarian point of view: I achieved what I had set out to do, but it was a calculating, dispiriting business, and I produced little of lasting consequence.

Although I didn't add in any meaningful way to the body of scientific knowledge, I learned a lot about how medical research works. Few, if any, researchers were inspired by scientific curiosity; the senior academics I encountered were motivated mainly by things like promotion, grant money, publications and merit awards. A medical research laboratory is a factory, which produces the raw material of data. From these data, many things may be fashioned: presentations to conferences, publications in journals, doctoral degrees, successful grant applications, even air miles. What went on in the nearby wards seemed of little consequence, apart from being a source of the bodily fluids ('clinical material') from which the data emerged. The academic Brahminate – the professors, heads of departments and deans – held great power over appointments, even to posts with little or no academic component. They sat on committees. They doled out the grant money to each other. Their clinical commitment was very often a sinecure, as NHS teaching hospitals were largely run in those days by very experienced 'junior' doctors. Senior registrars, particularly in surgery, were often approaching forty by the time they were appointed as consultants. These senior registrars were commonly more clinically capable and astute than the consultants, particularly the academic ones. One academic consultant physician I knew conducted a ward round once a week. His decisions were so bizarre, dangerous and reliably wrong that the ward sister and senior registrar had to conduct a 'real' round after they had first guided this buffoon around all the patients in a kind of Potemkin charade. Another academic – a surgeon – was so dangerous in the operating theatre that he was promoted to a professorship with mainly teaching duties to keep him away from patients. The dependable presence of the senior registrars left the Brahmins free to pursue the research game. They generally recruited to their ranks people of similar outlook and temperament, so the system was self-perpetuating.

I fell in with a gang of medical research fellows, and we met most lunchtimes in the doctors' dining room (the hospital still had one in the late 1980s), and, on Fridays, at the pub. We anxiously compared our progress in presentations to conferences and papers accepted for publication. All of them are now professors of greater or lesser eminence; two have become deans of medical schools. I cannot recall a single conversation about science: all we talked about was our careers. Genetics was the fashionable way to go into medical research in the late 1980s, and the research fellows were much occupied by this. Those who got into genetics early were racing ahead and were awash with grant money.

A venerable and eminent professor of medicine with whom I had worked was replaced by a geneticist with little in the way of clinical experience. This appointment was symbolic of the cultural shift in academic medicine. Up to that point, a professor of medicine was a sort of first among equals: he – it was usually he – had to command the respect of his colleagues as a clinician, was expected to take a lead in the teaching of medical students, and, if time permitted, to carry out research. By the late 1980s and early 1990s, this model was discarded, ushering in a new breed of senior academic, whose main role was the generation of grant money for laboratory research. They were invariably molecular biologists – geneticists or experts in some other aspect of basic cellular science, such as cytokine immunology. This new breed delegated teaching to more junior colleagues, and did little or no clinical work. The geneticist new-model professor of medicine of my acquaintance proudly abjured *all* clinical work, and his career peaked with a knighthood. David Sackett, founding father of evidence-based medicine, wrote in the *British Medical Journal* in 2004: 'Basic medical scientists have hijacked the granting bodies and have erected research policies that place greater value in serving their own personal curiosities than in serving the sick.' Nearly all senior academic appointments went to this new type of doctor, and the gulf between practising clinicians and researchers grew ever wider.

I do not regret the time I spent as a researcher. I had the outsider's perspective, but the insider's access. I was sometimes so emotionally detached from the activity that I felt like an anthropologist, conducting field studies on the behaviour of medical academics. Harry Collins, a sociologist of science, and an expert on expertise, carried out such anthropological studies on gravitational-wave physicists, and liked them: 'They're my ideal kind of academic. They're doing a slightly crazy, almost impossible project, and they're doing it for purely academic reasons with no economic payoff.' Collins's tame physicists embodied the lofty ideals of science, such as honesty, integrity, universalism, a willingness to expose one's ideas to the scrutiny of others and disinterestedness. I found little such idealism in my observations of medical researchers.

Towards the end of my time as a research fellow, I had a strange, post-modern, *Truman Show* experience. I was browsing at a book fair when I came across a short novel called *The Greatest Breakthrough since Lunchtime*. The author – a doctor – wrote under the pen name Colin Douglas, and the book was first published in 1977. The inner flap of the dust jacket leaves us in no doubt as to the saucy 1970s tone of this slim volume, with a photograph of a bespectacled young woman opening her doctor's white coat, to reveal that she is topless. The blurb promises 'a novel about idleness, promiscuity, drunkenness, boredom, adultery and medical research'. The hero, David Campbell, is a young doctor working in the Edinburgh teaching hospitals, and clearly based on the author himself. The novel is a period piece, of interest only to doctors who have trained or worked in Edinburgh, but I bought it out of curiosity. As I read it, I felt an unsettling familiarity with the scenes that Douglas describes. After house jobs, the hero drifts into a research fellowship, funded by a drug company, supervised by an academic physician called Rosamund Fyvie. Fyvie gives him the exact same pep talk as I received: 'She had suggested a basic method for the colonic mucosa experiment and told him about the lab where it might be done. He should "just play around with it for a day or two" and "read himself into the field" over the first week.' Many of the senior doctors in the book were clearly recognizable, even to an outsider like me. Campbell is set to work on 'faecal vitamins', not a million miles away from my whole gut lavage fluid antibodies. Douglas captures the boredom of this work well. As instructed, Campbell goes to the medical library to 'read himself into the field': 'As a second-rate cathedral might be at a similar hour of the day, the library was thinly populated, similarly by a selection of the most faithful and the most idle in the community... There was a girl who produced endless publications on mouse prostaglandins as though by a strange compulsion...'

Campbell seems to spend most of his time planning his next sexual conquest. Douglas describes Campbell's encounters with a nurse ('they liked each other, and sex together was marvellous') and an obliging lab technician ('"Christ, I needed that", said Lorna'). He becomes very quickly disillusioned with life as a researcher; his boss Fyvie is 'a raging psychopath on the make', and her senior registrar Dempster 'a dilettante con-man'. He muses on the motivation of his boss with his (married) colleague and love interest Jean:

> 'We're all in the business of helping to make her a professor. People and patients.' Campbell smiled like a wicked uncle. 'And that, my dear children, is the meaning of medical research.'
>
> Jean made a face and said, 'And what are you doing in it? Do you want to be a professor in the nineteen nineties?'
>
> 'I don't think I do. I can't make up my mind whether it's because I'm not nasty enough or because I don't care enough.'

The book ends with the death of a young girl with Down's syndrome (called a 'mongol' in the novel). She had been recruited, without her consent, by Dempster and Fyvie to a trial of an experimental drug for peptic ulcer, and dies as a result of bone-marrow failure caused by this agent. As I read this scene, I thought of my coeliac patient who had died after being recruited to the fatuous and futile drug trial which paid my wages. At the end of *The Greatest Breakthrough since Lunchtime*, Campbell abandons his research post and returns to clinical work.

How could this would-be titillating, trashy book, published more than ten years before, capture, with some accuracy, the flavour of my life as a research fellow? The novel – a bizarre hybrid of *Confessions of a House Officer* and sub-Illichian critique of medical research – crystallized some of my hard-earned lessons. Medical research was a Byzantine game played by cynical careerists; data were more important than ideas; professorships were more important than patients.

3

FIFTY GOLDEN YEARS

During the three years I spent as a research fellow, I presented my work to medical conferences, usually at the annual meeting of the British Society of Gastroenterology (BSG). Britain then led the world in this field, and the BSG was at the zenith of its influence, attracting thousands of delegates from all over the world to its meetings. If your paper was accepted, it would be either as a 'poster' or an 'oral' presentation. A poster presentation was less prestigious: all you had to do was stand, for a few hours, next to a board with your research findings pinned to it, and answer questions from anybody who happened to pass by and show an interest. Sometimes, nobody even looked at your poster, much less engaged you in scientific disputation. The oral presentations were a different event. These sessions were gladiatorial affairs, where the society's grandees attempted to outdo each other in rudeness towards the terrified presenters. (These grandees all looked like the more aristocratic members of Margaret Thatcher's cabinet, men like Lord Carrington and Douglas Hurd.) Such bullying was never questioned or challenged. It was taken for granted that one would be savaged by the big beasts at these presentations, particularly if one of them held a personal grudge against your boss. All of this was accepted as part of the rough and tumble of medical research, and was thought to toughen up the young. The 'plenary' or 'keynote' lectures were often given by basic scientists who delivered long and mainly incomprehensible talks on their subject to an audience composed mainly of clinical backwoodsmen who had little interest in such matters and who, after a boozy few days, returned no wiser or better informed to their district general hospitals and to the mundane business of treating the sick.

In September 1987, shortly after I moved to Edinburgh, the BSG held its golden jubilee meeting in London, marking fifty years since its foundation. A paper I submitted had been accepted as a poster presentation, so I travelled south to stand by my presentation in a vast hall in the University of London. This poster described some rather pedestrian research on coeliac disease I had conducted back in Ireland, and attracted little attention, except for a dismissive scowl from a senior academic I recognized as a leader in the field. The BSG was founded in 1937 by Sir Arthur Hurst (who had been knighted earlier that year) and was initially called the

Gastroenterological Club. Two of the society's senior members, John Alexander-Williams and Hugh Baron, wrote:

> The society, as we know it today, began its life essentially as a club for physicians and gentlemen. Members maintained exclusive standards by selecting only those of like mind and manners. 'Bounders' were denied membership by 'black-balling'. They embraced gastronomy as well as gastroenterology and the early meetings were characterized by their indulgence in good food and wine. As gentlemen, they championed modesty and eschewed publicity; their proceedings and papers were not published.

Had he been a gastroenterologist, Evelyn Waugh might have applied for membership of this club, which devoted much discussion to matters such as the wearing of formal dress at its dinners. The barbarians, however, were at the gates. During the 1950s and 1960s, the club became a society and admitted anyone keen to join, including foreign trainees and non-medical scientists: 'the British Society of Gastroenterology had become a society of scientists rather than a club for gentlemen', lamented Baron and Alexander Williams. Membership grew from 40 to 1,500. Two large meetings were needed every year to accommodate the number of scientific papers submitted. The pharmaceutical and medical devices industries partly funded these conferences, with huge exhibitions to promote their wares.

Thousands of delegates attended the golden jubilee meeting of 1987, and a huge hall accommodated the Trade Exhibition. Although the grandees didn't realize it, this meeting coincided with the end of British medicine's golden age. In the fifty years since Sir Arthur Hurst and his chums had gathered for a congenial dinner at the Langham Hotel in London, medicine had been transformed, and Britain was at the heart of this revolution. Sir Francis Avery Jones, grandest of the grandees, and, by common consent, the 'Father' of British Gastroenterology, had attended the first meeting in 1937, and was guest of honour in 1987. In those fifty years, Sir Francis had witnessed the arrival of penicillin, effective drug therapy for tuberculosis, kidney dialysis, organ transplantation, endoscopy, CT and MRI scanning, in vitro fertilization, the eradication of smallpox and the discovery of the double helix of DNA. Every delegate at the golden jubilee meeting was given a copy of a book (paid for and published by the drug company Smith, Kline & French) containing a selection of the most influential gastroenterology papers published in the previous half-century. The book's introduction was written, naturally, by Sir Francis, whose career had spanned this golden age.

This book tells the story of how medical research in Britain evolved over those fifty years, from curiosity-driven inquiry by passionate individuals to an industrialized, institutionalized activity. Many of the early papers from the 1940s and 1950s were written by single authors – single authorship of 'original' research papers is now almost unheard of, most being attributed to a committee of a dozen or more contributors. Most of these craggy individualists were full-time clinicians, not laboratory researchers, amateurs in the true sense of the word. Many of the publications in the collection evince a warm glow of nostalgia, a longing for simpler times. A paper by Sir Francis Avery Jones (single author), published in the *British Medical Journal* in 1943, describes the contemporary treatment of bleeding peptic (gastric and duodenal) ulcers. The main treatment in Sir Francis's day was diet: 'The patients received two-hourly purée feeds.' The contents, and sequence, of this diet are described in some detail: 'Cup of milky tea; three slices of thin bread-and-butter; bramble jelly; sponge cake.' His patients must have felt entirely safe in his patrician hands. The collection included the famous paper on Munchausen's syndrome by Sir Francis's old friend Richard Asher, his colleague at the Central Middlesex Hospital. Asher was a general physician who achieved some fame for his elegant, often contrary, essays. The type of glutinous prose found in medical journals has been labelled by Michael O'Donnell, the writer, doctor and broadcaster, as 'decorated municipal gothic', but in those innocent days of the early 1950s, journals like the *Lancet* published prose stylists like Asher. Munchausen's syndrome is a factitious disorder: those affected feign illness to gain attention. Asher named it after the fictional German noble-man: 'Like the famous Baron von Munchausen, the persons affected have always travelled widely; and their stories, like

those attributed to him, are both dramatic and untruthful.'
I find his assumption that the readers of the *Lancet* would be
familiar with R. E. Raspe's *Singular Travels, Campaigns and
Adventures of Baron Munchausen* strangely touching.

British science has a reputation for being at the forefront
of innovation, but of failing to put in the boring work of
practical application and commercial development. Such was
the history of endoscopy. Harold Hopkins was a physicist
based at Imperial College in London who discovered how to
convey optical images along flexible glass fibres. He had been
prompted to work on this after a chance meeting in 1951, at
a dinner party, with Hugh Gainsborough, a physician at St
George's Hospital. Gainsborough knew that Hopkins specialized in optics – he had invented the zoom lens – and suggested to him that he should try to develop a flexible endoscope.
At that time, endoscopes were rigid instruments, with very
limited views; 'intubation' – passing the instrument down
the patient's throat – was both dangerous (the pharynx or
oesophagus might be perforated) and extremely uncomfortable. Hopkins wrote a paper for *Nature* (the most prestigious of all science journals) in 1954, which is included in the
BSG's jubilee collection. He described a unit consisting of 'a
bundle of fibres of glass, or other transparent material, and
it therefore appears appropriate to introduce the term "fibrescope" to denote it'. Hopkins tried, and failed, to interest an
industrial partner. An enterprising South African gastroenterologist called Basil Hirschowitz, who had trained with

Sir Francis Avery Jones, picked up on Hopkins's idea, and along with two physicists at the University of Michigan, and with the financial support of the giant American Cystoscope Makers Inc (ACMI), developed the first commercial fibre-optic endoscope in 1960. Hirschowitz somehow managed to pass the endoscope down his own throat, before trying it out on a patient. The BSG awards an annual prize for innovation in endoscopy, named after Hopkins.

Although the British ceded commercial development of endoscopy to the Americans and the Japanese, they continued to come up with innovative applications of the new technology. In 1972, Peter Cotton, then a senior registrar at St Thomas' Hospital in London, wrote a paper for the *Lancet* describing how the common bile duct (which drains bile from the liver into the intestine) could be cannulated with an endoscope, and X-rays of this duct obtained by injecting dye. Bile duct obstruction due to gallstones and cancer is common, causing pain and jaundice. The procedure is called 'Endoscopic Retrograde Cholangio-Pancreatography' (ERCP) and is now routine. I have performed thousands. As well as identifying the cause of bile duct obstruction, it is used to relieve this obstruction by removing gallstones and inserting stents through blockages caused by cancers. Before ERCP, patients with bile duct obstruction had to undergo a major operation. Cotton was not the first to describe this technique; he went to Japan in 1971, where he spent three weeks with the gastroenterologist Kazuei Ogoshi, and brought the procedure back to Britain. He singlehandedly established ERCP in Britain, and trained the first generation of specialists who spread the procedure throughout Britain and North America. All British users of this procedure can trace their training, in a form of apostolic succession, back to Cotton. Despite this achievement, he failed to be appointed to a consultant post at St Thomas', an example, surely, of the British medical establishment's distrust of show-offs. He was later successful in his application for a post at the Middlesex Hospital, following which he was taken in hand by Sir Francis Avery Jones, an episode which he describes in his memoir *The Tunnel at the End of the Light*: 'Avery was kind to me when I was appointed to The Middlesex. He took me to lunch at the Athenaeum, the quintessential private London club, and explained some of the facts of private practice to me over roast pheasant and a frisky claret.'

Peptic ulceration is the theme of more than a quarter of all the papers in the jubilee collection. In the early decades of the twentieth century, up to 10 per cent of the adult male population in Britain were afflicted with chronic peptic ulcer. The disease was then commonly attributed to stress, a notion mocked by Richard Asher: 'One might just as well argue that the use of wrist watches was becoming increasingly common compared with Victorian times, and that therefore the increasing incidence of peptic ulcer was attributable to the wearing of wrist watches.' Many patients with peptic ulcer underwent major surgery. The work of the great Viennese surgeon Theodor Billroth (1829–94) began the development of a variety of operations for ulcer disease, and this type of surgery made up most of the workload of abdominal surgeons in the first half of the twentieth century. Some of these operations were so 'radical' that the treatment was often worse than the disease, creating a whole population of patients known as 'gastric cripples' who suffered ever after from emaciation and malabsorption.

By the early 1970s, the pharmaceutical industry was becoming increasingly influential in medical research. James (later Sir James) Black of Smith, Kline & French's Research Institute described the histamine H_2-receptor in the stomach in a paper published in *Nature* in 1972 and included in the collection. This receptor controls acid secretion in the stomach. Black developed a drug to block the receptor, thus reducing acid secretion. Cimetidine (branded as 'Tagamet' by Smith, Kline & French) was the first effective drug treatment for peptic ulcer, and the first so-called 'blockbuster' drug. This success was the model for later, even more profitable, blockbusters, the spectacular profits from which created the global giant which is now Big Pharma. Although cimetidine *did* heal ulcers, patients invariably relapsed once the course of treatment was completed, so most continued taking the drug indefinitely. Cimetidine was certainly an advance, but not a cure. Paradoxically, this limitation was the key to its commercial success, and the reason why it became the first blockbuster drug: because so many patients took the drug for years – rather than weeks – sales were huge. Smith, Kline & French made a fortune, and Sir James Black won the Nobel Prize for Medicine in 1988.

Sir Francis Avery Jones celebrated the great progress made in the half-century of the speciality, but lamented the failures in other areas:

> Although remarkable progress has been achieved in these fifty years, there are still many unsolved problems. The clinical study of diseases, their diagnosis and treatment has made giant strides forward, but unfortunately the causes of major illnesses, including peptic ulcer, ulcerative colitis and Crohn's disease, still remain to be discovered.

Sir Francis was seventy-seven when he wrote his introduction to this selection of papers, so perhaps cannot be blamed for not keeping a close eye on the medical literature. Had he done so, he might have spotted that for five years running up to the jubilee meeting in 1987, Robin Warren (a pathologist) and Barry Marshall (a trainee gastroenterologist) from Perth, Australia, had produced several papers strongly suggesting that peptic ulcer and gastritis were caused by a bacterium called *Helicobacter pylori*. Less than two months after the jubilee meeting, the *Lancet* published a paper by a Dublin group led by Colm O'Morain, which showed that eradication of *Helicobacter* not only healed duodenal ulcers, but crucially – and unlike cimetidine – kept them healed. Marshall and

Warren published a paper a year later, also in the *Lancet*, with the same conclusion. A combination of antibiotics taken for a week was shown to cure a condition which up to then very often required a mutilating surgical procedure. It is not difficult to understand, therefore, why the global gastroenterology community might have felt a collective cognitive dissonance. Many initially ignored it, but by the early 1990s, most were convinced. The whole clinical and academic infrastructure which had grown around the surgical treatment of peptic ulcer simply disappeared, and the surgeons found other things to do.

Arthur Hedley Visick, surgeon at York County Hospital, might also have experienced severe cognitive dissonance had he survived into the late 1980s. He wrote a paper for the *Lancet* in 1948 on 'Measured Radical Gastrectomy', a procedure he performed on 500 patients between 1936 and 1947: the operation removed between one-half and two-thirds of the stomach in patients with chronic peptic ulcer. Surgeons travelled to York from all over Britain and abroad to watch Visick operate. He died of a stroke in 1949 at the age of fifty-one, having collapsed in the surgical outpatients. Visick did not survive long enough to be told that all of those 500 patients could have been cured with a course of antibiotics. The *Helicobacter* story, however, is not a simple narrative of the plucky Australian outsiders taking on a monolithic medical establishment. *Helicobacter* became the centre of a new medical industry, just as gastric acid secretion was the obsession of a previous generation. *Helicobacter* got its own conferences and journals; Marshall and Warren won the Nobel Prize for Medicine in 2005, and many others further down the food chain got chairs and large research grants. The Gadarene researchers who once followed the dogma of gastric acid secretion now switched allegiance to *Helicobacter*. Few admitted that peptic ulcers were already in steep decline by the time *Helicobacter* was discovered, and that most such ulcers were by then caused by anti-inflammatory painkillers (including aspirin), not *Helicobacter*. The great majority of people infected with *Helicobacter* never develop a peptic ulcer; eradicating the organism in those without ulcer is of questionable benefit. In developing countries such as India, the vast majority of the population is infected with *Helicobacter*, yet peptic ulcer is rare. No matter. The *Helicobacter* bandwagon drove on regardless, with the new dogma proclaimed by consensus conferences, and, when I checked on PubMed this morning, 40,580 publications. I am a co-author of one of these 40,580 papers. An enterprising researcher from an institution in another city invited me to collaborate on a study of the prevalence of *Helicobacter* infection in patients with coeliac disease, for no other reason than he had a blood test for *Helicobacter* and I had a large bank of stored blood from coeliac patients. There was no interesting question to answer, and I don't think we found very much, but we did get a publication out of it. This paper is a good example of the man-with-a-hammer scientific opportunism. There was no plausible biological reason why *Helicobacter* and coeliac disease should have any connection, and the question was of little interest either clinically or scientifically. And yet: a paper was published.

Many of the papers in the BSG collection describe work and ideas which are now discredited. Medical research is a conformist activity, driven largely by received opinion. The collective obsession with the physiology of gastric acid secretion is now perplexing, particularly when the (admittedly counter-intuitive) answer (*Helicobacter*) was knocking loudly at the door. Long before Marshall and Warren discovered *Helicobacter*, papers had appeared intermittently in the journals describing bacteria in the stomach, but were dismissed on the grounds that bacteria could not possibly survive in the acid environment of the stomach. Alan Bennett once wrote about his uncle Norris, who was obsessed by his firm conviction that arthritis could be cured by the simple expedient of cutting off the feet of one's socks. Perhaps the medical establishment thought that the idea of curing peptic ulcer with a course of antibiotics was about as biologically plausible as Uncle Norris's cure for arthritis. Many of these important discoveries – again, *Helicobacter* – were often serendipitous findings by enthusiasts with prepared minds, rather than the result of planned, lavishly funded institutional research. Diseases come and go, and effective treatments often arise when the disease was declining anyway (peptic ulcer, tuberculosis). Today's exciting innovation is tomorrow's stifling consensus, while other once-exciting innovations will tomorrow be as forgotten as Ozymandias, King of Kings. Since 1987, Big Science has taken over, and the jubilee papers now seem quaint and almost innocent.

Why had so much progress been made during this fifty-year period? The Second World War drove technological innovation; the post-war years saw a dramatic expansion of academic medicine and biomedical research, particularly in the US. Vannevar Bush's 1945 report, *Science: the Endless Frontier*, set the agenda for biomedical research. Bush, formerly dean of engineering at MIT, chaired the National Defense Research Council, which was established by President Roosevelt in 1940. Roosevelt recognized that science had been crucial to the war effort and wanted the lessons learned to be applied to the development of science in peacetime. Bush's report emphasized the primacy of 'basic' research and government funding. The report led to a huge expansion in scientific research at American universities and a tenfold increase in government funding from the 1940s to the 1960s. Universities, which until then saw their main function as teaching, became the principal location of scientific research. The concentration on 'basic' science was not universally welcomed. The great epidemiologist and clinician Alvan Feinstein wrote in 1987: 'The research changed its orientation. The pre-clinical sciences became detached from their clinical origins and were converted into "basic biomedical sciences" with goals that... often had no overt relationship to clinical phenomena.'

Following the foundation of the NHS, there was a major expansion of academic medicine in Britain and the establishment of research-focused teaching hospitals, such as the Royal Postgraduate Medical School (RPMS) at the Hammersmith Hospital. The 1944 *Goodenough Report on Medical Education* recommended that 'every medical school should be a university medical school'. This led to a dramatic expansion in the number of academic medical posts, with the creation of more than fifty new clinical professorships. After the war, the RPMS set the agenda for British medical research; the consultants there were not allowed to engage in private practice, and they were essentially full-time clinical researchers. Clinical research was then unhampered by bureaucracy. This came with a downside: many patients were abused – unaware that they were being used as guinea pigs, they underwent invasive and dangerous procedures purely for research purposes, without their knowledge or consent. Sir John McMichael was director of the Hammersmith school for twenty years after the war; he pioneered the techniques of cardiac catheterization and liver biopsy, both now routine procedures. In the early 1950s, Alex Paton, then a registrar at the Hammersmith, kept a private diary in which he expressed his concerns: 'We and anyone else at Hammersmith use subjects for experiments who will not necessarily benefit by them... The beds are really nothing more than an annexe to the medical laboratories.' The physician Maurice Pappworth drew the public's attention to these unethical practices in

1967 with his book *Human Guinea Pigs*, and for his trouble was ostracized by the medical establishment. Writing on McMichael's experiments on cardiac catheterization in elderly patients with heart failure, Pappworth wrote: 'It appears that doctors sometimes forget that those who are most in need of help, sympathy and gentle treatment are not the less sick but the most sick, and that among these the dying and the old have pre-eminent claims.' Professor (later Dame) Sheila Sherlock was a protégée of McMichael's at the Hammersmith, and later Professor of Medicine at the Royal Free Hospital. Neither cultivated a bedside manner; Sherlock's *British Medical Journal* obituary stated that 'there was little place for good taste or patients' feelings'. Pappworth wrote a letter to the *Lancet* in 1955, in which he referred to Sherlock's 'dastardly experiments' and accused British teaching hospitals of being 'dominated by ghoulish physiologists masquerading as clinicians'. The *Lancet* declined to publish.

Sheila Sherlock's protégé – and later rival – Roger Williams set up the Liver Unit at King's College Hospital, which became the largest such unit in Britain. Working with Roy Calne, a surgeon at Addenbrooke's Hospital in Cambridge, Williams established liver transplantation in Britain. They wrote up their initial experience in the *British Medical Journal* in 1969, describing the outcome of transplantation in thirteen patients. Only two of the thirteen survived to four months; four died within thirty-six hours of the operation. Many others might have given up at this point, but Williams and Calne kept going. They learned how to prevent rejection of the transplanted organ with new drugs to suppress the body's immune system; they refined pre- and post-operative care; they established which diseases could be successfully treated by transplantation, and thus improved the selection of patients. Liver transplantation is now a successful and routine treatment, carried out in several British hospitals, and the vast majority of patients survive. Were the *British Medical Journal* to publish a paper now with these mortality figures, the doctors involved would be ordered by their managers to desist, and might well find themselves before the General Medical Council.

The British medical establishment resisted the foundation of the NHS, and Aneurin Bevan had to offer generous inducements to the hospital consultants to ensure their cooperation. He allowed them to continue practising privately, and also introduced the financial incentives called merit awards. From 1948 to sometime in the late 1970s, these consultants enjoyed professional and academic freedoms that today's beleaguered doctors can only dream of. Peter Cotton described the gentlemanly pace of his colleagues in the mid-1970s: 'Many of my consultant colleagues seemed to spend most of their time up the street in private practice, allowing their chauffeurs to take them to the Middlesex twice a week for a ward round and a pot of tea with the ward sister.' Many, if not most, contented themselves with Harley Street and the assignation for tea with sister, but the enthusiasts were free to pursue their obsessions. Cotton wrote admiringly of his senior colleague at the Middlesex, Peter Ball:

> He worked two days a week at the hospital, one day at Kew gardens where he was revising the taxonomy of Orchids, one day in private practice, and one at the London Zoo, where he did research on snakes and various parasites. Part of his research with worms took him regularly to Africa, and he actually imported some specimens by swallowing them.

British medicine's prestige rose dramatically during the three decades after the Second World War, and research was producing treatments that were demonstrably and dramatically effective. Consultants – particularly those based in the great teaching hospitals – enjoyed almost complete professional and academic freedom. They answered neither to administrators nor to the general public. Their eccentricities and scientific passions were not only tolerated, but actively encouraged. Many, as Peter Cotton noted, abused this freedom to make money, but others, such as his colleague Peter Ball – and Cotton himself – pursued loftier ambitions. Cotton had established ERCP, a major new technique, when he was still – technically – a trainee (senior registrar). This would now be unthinkable. By the mid-1980s, Cotton had a global reputation, and doctors came from all over the world to learn ERCP at his unit in the Middlesex Hospital. He had, however, become disenchanted with the NHS. The hospital, operating on a fixed annual budget, was not impressed by the fame of their young star gastroenterologist, and the many overseas trainees he attracted, and once sent him written instructions 'to do 25 per cent less procedures next year'. The final straw came when the hospital told him they would no longer allow the overseas trainees to work there (even though they were unpaid) 'because they attracted patients who they had to feed and bathe'. In 1986, Cotton was appointed Chief of Endoscopy at Duke University in North Carolina, and spent the remainder of his career in the US.

Power in medicine slowly shifted from the teaching-hospital clinician-aristocrats – doctors like Sir Francis Avery Jones – to the new laboratory-based professional researchers, the Big Science Brahmins. The historian Roy Porter wrote in 1997:

> Today, though one or two transplant surgeons are house-hold names, the real medical power lies in the hands of Nobel Prize-winning researchers, the presidents of the great medical schools, and the boards of multi-billion dollar hospital conglomerates, health maintenance organizations and pharmaceutical companies.

The great teaching hospitals are now run by managers, and the consultants, although their number has increased dramatically since the mid-1980s, are collectively and individually without influence. Doctors still receive knighthoods and damehoods, but they are bestowed mainly on the academic Brahminate and the committee men and women. I last attended a BSG meeting in Manchester in 2014; the clinician-aristocrats had disappeared. In their place was a collection of demoralized Stakhanovite workers, none of whom had ever lunched at the Athenaeum over roast pheasant and a frisky claret. The golden age had passed.

4

BIG BAD SCIENCE

The professionalization, industrialization and globalization of medical research was well under way by the time of the BSG's Golden Jubilee Meeting in 1987, and by the 2000s, the process was complete. From the 1950s to the 1990s, many NHS teaching-hospital consultants carried out significant research, even though they had no formal academic appointment. In the new millennium, this all changed. In the wake of the scandal at Alder Hey Hospital in Liverpool (where the organs of children who had died at the hospital had been retained, for research purposes, without the parents' knowledge or consent), the bureaucracy around medical research grew to the point where only full-time research professionals, supported by a secretariat to handle all the red tape, could do it. The Thatcher-era health reforms disempowered hospital consultants, who now found themselves at the clinical coalface, at the beck and call of managers: with so many targets to reach, there was no time for research. The academic Brahminate withdrew ever more from the hospitals. Teaching was taken over by specialists in medical education, allowing the researchers to concentrate entirely on grant applications and committee work. The dividing line between academic medicine and industry became so blurred as to be almost invisible.

The phrase 'Big Science' was coined by the physicist Alvin Weinberg to mean the type of science that is laboratory-based, lavishly funded and conducted in large, usually university-based research facilities, overseen by powerful, quasi-feudal, academic managerialists. The research industry draws in vast quantities of public money, and sells itself to politicians and industry as a driver of economic growth. The molecular biologists often use the hackneyed and pompous phrase 'from bench to bedside' to boost their claim that their labours are relevant to real-life patients. Although this type of research has grown massively since the late 1980s, advances which benefit patients have been modest and unspectacular compared to the golden age. The Big Science Brahmins are now so removed from the clinical front line that the phrase rings hollow. The basic science model seems superficially plausible. It is based on the Cartesian idea of the body as an elaborate machine; disease is a malfunction of this machine. To cure disease, you must first understand how the machine works. A 2003 study from John Ioannidis showed the limitations of such 'mechanistic' research. Ioannidis is a Greek–American professor of medicine at Stanford Medical School, and is the founder and leader of a new discipline known as 'meta-research', or research about research. He and his wife Despina – a paediatrician – examined 101 basic science discoveries, published in the top basic science journals (*Science*, *Nature*, *Cell*, etc.) between 1979 and 1983, all of which claimed to have a clinical application. Twenty years later, twenty-seven of these technologies had been tested clinically, five eventually were approved for marketing, of which only one was deemed to have clinical benefit.

Most of the diseases that kill us now are caused by, and associated with, ageing. We just wear out. Dementia, heart disease, stroke and cancer kill us now, not smallpox and Spanish flu. Medicine can still pull off spectacular rescues of mortally sick young people, but these triumphs are notable for their relative rarity. The other flaw in the Big Science theory is that a great deal of what is laid at medicine's door to fix has nothing to do with malfunction of the machine; much of the work of GPs is helping people cope not with disease but with living problems, or 'shit life syndrome', as some call it. More than 50 per cent of my outpatients have symptoms caused by psychosomatic conditions, such as irritable bowel syndrome, which cannot be elucidated or cured by the molecular biologists. Humans have always experienced stress and distress, but only in the twentieth century did we (at least those of us living in rich countries) decide that the inevitable vicissitudes of living should be reconfigured as medical problems.

Does medicine still need breakthroughs? Is research still worth doing? Medicine should try its utmost to prevent *premature* mortality; I would arbitrarily set this as anything below eighty. More importantly, medicine should deal better with pain, suffering and disability. I do not believe, however, that better ways of relieving suffering will emerge from molecular medicine. There is a philosophical, moral and existential paradox at the heart of research. Death is the inevitable product of disease, ageing and the body's breakdown. Research aims to 'fight' this, yet we accept, deep within our being, that death is not only inevitable, it is *good*. Why, then, should we continue to fight this unwinnable and unnecessary battle? *Premature* mortality has declined dramatically and is now rare; most of us can expect to live into our eighth or ninth decade. Extending longevity beyond that is misguided and dangerous. The dramatic increase in human longevity witnessed in the twentieth century is so new and so dramatic that as a species we haven't learned how to deal with it.

What, then, should medical research do? The Big Science model – find the 'cause' and thence the 'cure' – should still be applied to some diseases. Crohn's disease (a chronic inflammatory disorder of the intestine), for example, causes long-term disability in a predominantly young patient population, and often requires permanent treatment with dangerous immunosuppressive drugs. A cure would be an unquestioned benefit. Research, unfortunately, will never help most of what ails mankind: growing old and dying. These are eternal human verities, but we expect medicine to somehow solve this riddle. Epidemiologists and public health doctors would argue that medicine now contributes little to health in developed countries, and that poverty, lack of education and deprivation are now the main drivers of poor health. This is almost certainly true. Although vaccination and antibiotics contributed significantly to the increase in human longevity in the mid-twentieth century, medical care now has little direct influence on the health of a population, accounting for only about 10 per cent of variation. Furthermore, some have argued persuasively that if we were to simply apply evenly and logically what research has *already* proven, health care would be transformed.

Big Science has not delivered the breakthroughs expected of it, yet it consumes the great majority of medical research funding, so other, possibly more productive, types of research have been starved of resources. Why is this model a failure? As my experience of research taught me, Big Science is funded to produce data, rather than original ideas. The biophysicist John Platt wrote in *Science* in 1964: 'We speak piously of taking measurements and making small studies that will "add another brick to the temple of science". Most such bricks just lie around in the brickyard.' Another limitation of the Big Science model is its assumption that nothing unexpected is ever encountered, that research is something that is *planned*, yet many of the great scientific discoveries (penicillin, *Helicobacter*) were unanticipated and serendipitous.

The doctor and polemicist Bruce Charlton has observed that the culture of contemporary medical research is so conformist that truly original thinkers can no longer prosper in such an environment, and that science selects for perseverance and sociability at the expense of intelligence and creativity:

> Modern science is just too dull an activity to attract, retain or promote many of the most intelligent and creative people. In particular, the requirement for around 10, 15, or even 20 years of post-graduate 'training' before even having a chance at doing some independent research of one's own choosing, is enough to deter almost anyone with a spark of vitality or self-respect; and utterly exclude anyone with an urgent sense of vocation for creative endeavour. Even after a decade or two of 'training' the most likely scientific prospect is that of researching a topic determined by the availability of funding rather than scientific importance, or else functioning as a cog in someone else's research machine. Either way, the scientist will be working on somebody else's problem – not his own. Why would any serious intellectual wish to aim for such a career?

Charlton observed that modern medical research is a collective activity, requiring the co-ordination and co-operation of many sub-specialists: being a 'team-player' is an essential attribute for such work. He argues that the very best scientists are 'wasted as team players. The very best scientists can function only as mavericks because they are doing science for vocational reasons.' Charles Darwin, for example, worked alone, mainly at home, without a university appointment or funding. He had the good fortune of independent means, and worked only on subjects that stimulated his curiosity.

Big Science has a Big, Bad Secret: it doesn't work. This is down to a combination of perverse incentives, careerism and commercialization. The incentivization of bad science is nothing new. Donald T. Campbell, an American social scientist, coined his eponymous law in 1979: 'If researchers are incentivized to increase the number of papers published, they will modify their methods to produce the largest possible number of publishable results rather than the most rigorous investigations.' The medical statistician Douglas Altman wrote an editorial for the *British Medical Journal* in 1994 entitled 'The scandal of poor medical research'. This editorial won a 2015 poll of *BMJ* readers for the paper the journal should be most proud of publishing. Altman simply articulated clearly and concisely what everyone within academic medicine knew:

Put simply, much poor research arises because researchers feel compelled for career reasons to carry out research that they are ill equipped to perform, and nobody stops them. Regardless of whether a doctor intends to pursue a career in research, he or she is usually expected to carry out research with the aim of publishing several papers.

... The poor quality of much medical research is widely acknowledged, yet disturbingly the leaders of the medical profession seem only minimally concerned about the problem and make no apparent efforts to find a solution... The issue here is not one of statistics as such. Rather it is a more general failure to appreciate the basic principles underlying scientific research, coupled with the 'publish or perish' climate... We need less research, better research, and research done for the right reasons.

Over the past few years, Big Scientists have become increasingly concerned by what they call 'the Replication Crisis': the indisputable fact that most research findings are never repeated – replicated – to confirm that the findings are real. Most 'positive' studies are never repeated to see if the finding withstands further scrutiny: less than 1 per cent of all psychological research, for example, is ever replicated. The Royal Society – the world's grandest scientific institution – produces an open-access online journal, *Royal Society Open Science*, which in 2016 published a paper entitled 'The natural selection of bad science' by Paul Smaldino (from the University of California) and Richard McElreath (from the

Max Planck Institute in Leipzig). Using a Darwinian model of natural selection, the authors argued that Big Science is driven by multiple perverse incentives to produce bad work. Academic promotion in science depends very much on publication metrics, which are based on the overall number of papers, and how often these papers are cited by other researchers. These metrics encourage scientists to value quantity over quality. The rate of production of new scientific papers is increasing exponentially: global scientific output doubles every nine years. Most of the increase is driven by perverse incentives. Richard Horton, the editor of the *Lancet*, wrote: 'Part of the problem is that no one is incentivized to be right.'

The new breed of biomedical career researcher is often a great salesman for his work. Real scientists – like Harry Collins's particle wave physicists – tend to be reticent, self-effacing, publicity-shy and full of doubt and uncertainty, unlike the gurning hucksters who seem to infest medical research. Smaldino and McElreath wearily observed:

In the years between 1974 and 2014, the frequency of the words 'innovative', 'ground-breaking' and 'novel' in PubMed abstracts increased by 2,500 per cent or more. As it is unlikely that individual scientists have really become 25 times more innovative in the past 40 years, one can only conclude that this language evolution reflects a response to increasing pressures for novelty, and more generally to stand out from the crowd.

They argue 'that the incentives to generate a lengthy CV have particular consequences on the ecology of scientific communities'. Journals have a bias for 'positive' results: this incentivizes research techniques and statistics that have a high rate of false positives. The majority of the false positive publications are not due to deliberate fraud, but to practices such as 'p-hacking' – the common practice of putting raw data through statistical software until a 'significant' p-value is found. ('P' stands for probability: a p-value of 0.05 means that the probability of the result occurring by chance is 1 in 20; a p-value of 0.01 means the probability is 1 in 100, and so on. A p-value of 0.05 is regarded as the lowest level of statistical 'significance'.) 'P-hacking' is also known as 'data torture' and 'data dredging'. What is to be done? Smaldino and McElreath are not optimistic:

> Institutional change is difficult to accomplish, because it requires coordination on a large scale, which is often costly to early adopters. Yet such change is needed to ensure the integrity of science... A more drastic suggestion is to alter the fitness landscape entirely by changing the selection pressures: the incentives for success. This is likely to be quite difficult.

Big Science has recognized its big problem, and is trying – or knows that it is important to be *seen* to try – to fix it. In April 2015, a meeting was held at the Wellcome Trust in

London, under the collective auspices of the Academy of Medical Sciences, the Wellcome Trust, the Medical Research Council and the Biotechnology and Biological Sciences Research Council. This was called a 'Symposium on the Reproducibility and Reliability of Biomedical Research', which sounds distinctly bland, but the meeting was the first serious attempt to address the undisputed fact that medical research has lost its way. The meeting was a semi-secret affair, with attendees asked to observe Chatham House rules – that is, participants are free to use the information, but cannot identify the speaker or their affiliation. Those who worked for government agencies were particularly anxious not to be quoted. Richard Horton wrote in his own journal shortly after the symposium: 'Why the paranoid concern for secrecy and non-attribution? Because this symposium – on the reproducibility and reliability of biomedical research – touched on one of the most sensitive issues in science today: the idea that something has gone fundamentally wrong with one of our greatest human creations.'

The summary document of the meeting concluded that there is no single cause of irreproducibility. The factors they identified included: (1) p-hacking; (2) HARKing, short for Hypothesising After the Results are Known – inventing a plausible explanation for the result that was obtained, after the data have been inspected; (3) not publishing studies unless they have a 'significant' result; (4) lack of statistical power, i.e. recruiting so few subjects that it is impossible to tell if an effect is real; (5) technical errors; (6) inadequate description of experimental methods, such that other researchers cannot repeat the study; and (7) weak experimental design. They acknowledged that 'cultural factors, such as a highly competitive research environment and the high value placed on novelty and publication in high-profile journals, may also play a part'. How can all this be fixed? The eminent scientists who attended the meeting at the Wellcome Trust had some typically banal suggestions, such as 'providing further education in research methods for scientists', 'due diligence by bodies that fund research', and 'greater openness and transparency'.

It was inevitable with so many and such varied perverse incentives that outright fraud would become commonplace in medical research. Although only 2 per cent of researchers have admitted to falsifying data, the true figure is thought to be much higher. The website Retraction Watch tracks scientific papers which have been retracted or withdrawn by their authors for reasons of fraud or falsification. Dr Yoshitaka Fujii, a Japanese anaesthetist, is currently top of the Retraction Watch leaderboard with 183 retracted studies. Laypeople are especially shocked by scientific fraud: when Al Gore led a congressional inquiry into scientific fraud in 1981, the historian Daniel Kevles observed that 'for Gore and for many others, fraud in the biomedical sciences was akin to pederasty among priests'. Most doctors have come across scientific fraud, and are less shocked by it. I knew one researcher whose deliberate falsification of data was an open secret in the hospital where I then worked; his 'work' had been published in several major journals. A friend and colleague co-authored several of these papers. I told him about the researcher's methods, and was answered with a weary shrug. Deliberate fraud – so-called 'scientific pornography' – is indeed shocking, but is a minor problem compared to the combination of careerism, vested interest, self-deception and perverse incentives which creates so much bad science. Researchers are generally too careful and too cunning to carry out deliberate fraud when they can achieve the same result by other, less detectable means.

Medical journals are embedded in this problem. When I qualified, it was possible – just – for a diligent and disciplined doctor to keep up both with developments in medicine in general, and with their own speciality. One read the great general journals (the *Lancet, British Medical Journal* and *New England Journal of Medicine*), as well as perhaps two specialist journals. These journals then carried the authority of Moses' Tablets of Stone. Since then, the exponentially rising quantity of biomedical research output has to go somewhere, and that somewhere is a journal. The prestige of a journal is now based on a metric called the impact factor. The impact factor is calculated from the number of citations, received in that year, of articles published in that journal. The impact factor of the *New England Journal of Medicine*, for example, is 72.4, for the *Lancet* 44 and for the *Irish*

Medical Journal 0.31. The performance of medical academics is judged on metrics such as citation count and the h-index (calculated from the number of publications and number of citations of each paper). Inevitably, academics game these metrics. Goodhart's law (named after the British economist) states that once a variable is adopted as a policy target, it rapidly loses its ability to capture the phenomenon or characteristic that is supposedly being measured; adoption of a new indicator 'leads to changes in behaviour with gaming to maximize the score, perverse incentives, and unintended consequences'. Mario Biagioli, professor of law and of science and technology at the University of California, Davis, cited this law in an analysis of how individual researchers and institutions game bibliometric indices, such as impact factors, citation indices and rankings. This gaming has become increasingly sophisticated: one new wheeze is for researchers, when submitting a paper to a journal, to give the journal fake email addresses of potential 'reviewers'. (Journals send all submitted papers to be reviewed by experts in the field, a practice known as 'peer review'.) The authors then use these fake email addresses to supply flattering reviews back to the journal, thus increasing the chance of publication. In some universities – typically in emerging countries – researchers are unofficially obliged to cite the work of other researchers in the institution, to increase their 'citation index'. Biagioli concluded: 'The audit culture of universities – their love affair with metrics, impact factors, citation statistics and rankings – does not just incentivize this new form of bad behaviour. It enables it.'

When biomedical science expanded dramatically in the post-Second World War decades, so too did the number of journals available to publish all this new research. Scientific publishing has global revenues of more than £19 billion, placing it somewhere between the record and film industries in size. The profit margins of scientific publishers are greater than any of the tech giants: in 2010, Elsevier reported profits of £724 million on £2 billion in revenue, a margin of 36 per cent. Their business model is truly remarkable: the product (scientific papers) is given to them for free, and the purchasers of the product are mainly government-funded institutes and universities. In his brilliant 2017 *Guardian* essay 'Is the staggeringly profitable business of scientific publishing bad for science?' Stephen Buranyi wrote:

It is as if the *New Yorker* or the *Economist* demanded that journalists write and edit each other's work for free, and asked the government to foot the bill. Outside observers tend to fall into a sort of stunned disbelief when describing this setup. A 2004 parliamentary science and technology committee report on the industry drily observed that 'in a traditional market suppliers are paid for the goods they provide'. A 2005 Deutsche Bank report referred to it as a 'bizarre' 'triple-pay' system, in which 'the state funds most research, pays the salaries of most of those checking the quality of research, and then buys most of the published product'.

The person who did most to create this unbeatable business model was Robert Maxwell. Born Ján Hoch in what was then Czechoslovakia, he reinvented himself during the war as a British officer, and became the millionaire 'Robert Maxwell'. Immediately after the war, the British government decided that, although British science was exploding, its scientific journals were dismal. They chose to pair the British publisher Butterworths with the German publisher Springer, which was thought to have greater commercial expertise. At this time, Maxwell was shipping scientific articles to Britain on behalf of Springer. The Butterworths directors knew Maxwell, and hired him and a former spy, the Austrian metallurgist Paul Rosbaud. In 1951, Maxwell bought both Butterworths' and Springer's shares, and set up a new company which he called Pergamon. Rosbaud saw that new journals would be required to accommodate all the research produced in the post-war scientific boom. He hit on the simple but brilliant idea of persuading prominent academics that their field needed a new journal, and then installed the same prominent academics as the editors. Maxwell entertained the scientists at his Oxfordshire mansion, Headington Hill Hall; they were easily seduced. In 1959, Pergamon was publishing 40 journals; by 1965, the number rose to 150.

Maxwell understood that the business was almost limit-less. After Watson and Crick's discovery of the double-helix structure of DNA, he decided that the future was in bio-medical sciences. Maxwell called the business 'a perpetual financing machine'. Journals now set the agenda for science, and in the process researchers were incentivized to produce work that appealed to the journal editors, particularly the new, glamorous, high-impact basic science journals, such as *Cell*, *Nature* and *Science*. After Maxwell's mysterious death in 1991 – he fell overboard from his yacht – Pergamon and its 400 journals was bought by Elsevier. In the late 1990s, it was widely predicted that the Internet would make these companies obsolete, but Elsevier accommodated to the new reality by selling electronic access to its journals in bundles of hundreds. In 2015, the *Financial Times* labelled Elsevier 'the business the Internet could not kill'. Robert Maxwell correctly predicted in 1988 that in the future there would only be a handful of huge scientific publishing companies, who would operate in an electronic age with no printing or delivery costs, leading to almost 'pure profit'.

Maxwell would have admired the pure shamelessness of the 'predatory' journals. They emerged around ten years ago to meet the urgent need of researchers to get published – any-where. They will publish anything, as long as the authors pay. It has been estimated that there are now 8,000 such jour-nals, publishing 420,000 articles a year. I receive emails from them most days, inviting me to contribute, or to become a member of their editorial boards. The existence of this new thriving industry is the logical conclusion of the dominance of journals over scientists, and the prevailing culture of medical research. Nobody reads the predatory journals, but then, most articles in 'respectable' journals are also unread: half of all articles published are never cited. Richard Smith, who edited the *British Medical Journal* from 1991 to 2004, joked that the publishers of medical journals are like mustard manufacturers: they make their money from material that is never used.

Papers submitted to the 'respectable' journals are sent out for external peer review. There is a now a general consensus that this process is deeply flawed; most papers eventually find a home of greater or lesser prestige. If your paper is rejected, send it to another journal, and so on until one eventually publishes your work. Drummond Rennie, deputy editor of the influential *Journal of the American Medical Association*, wrote:

> There seems to be no study too fragmented, no hypothesis too trivial, no literature citation too biased or too egotistical, no design too warped, no methodology too bungled, no presentation of results too inaccurate, too obscure, and too contradictory, no analysis too self-serving, no argument too circular, no conclusions too trifling or too unjustified, and no grammar and syntax too offensive for a paper to end up in print.

Many researchers are in open revolt against the journals. They argue that all research should be published openly, online, with all the data available for inspection; all trial protocols should be similarly published, and all trials registered. More importantly, they argue, trial proposals should be scrutinized and need to pass some basic requirements to determine that they are useful, that they will answer a real question. Innovations such as Wellcome Open Research and F1000Research have shown the journals that scientists could run science publishing without them. Even Elsevier has concluded that the journal era is nearing an end: they now describe themselves as a 'Big Data Company', and a 'global information analytics business that helps institutions and professionals progress science, advance healthcare, and improve performance'. Elsevier is positioning itself to become the only company that sells publishing services such as software to scientists, becoming a force to rival Facebook or Google. Richard Smith warned: 'Elsevier will come to know more about the world's scientists – their needs, demands, aspirations, weaknesses, and buying patterns – than any other organization. The profits will come from those data and that knowledge. The users of Facebook are both the customers and the product, and scientists will be both the customers and the product of Elsevier.' But a revolt is already under way: Swedish and German universities cancelled their Elsevier subscriptions, and the website Sci-Hub, which Elsevier has sued, provides free access to 67 million research articles. The European Commission has called for full open access to all scientific publications by 2020, and has invited bids for the development of an EU-wide open-access science publishing platform, a move that has been criticized by Jon Tennant, a researcher working on public access to scientific knowledge, as 'finding new ways of channelling public money into private hands'. Many believe that the only way to sort this out is for the scientific community to take control of how their work is communicated.

John Ioannidis observed how perverse incentives, and the natural selection described by Smaldino and McElreath, have created a new breed of managerialist-scientist, whose success is measured, not by originality of thought, or new discoveries, but by volume of grant income generated, and PhD students and post-doctoral scientists (postdocs) employed:

> Of course, those who are the most successful in grants-manship include many superb scientists. However, they also include a large share (in many places, the majority) of the most aggressive, take-all, calculating managers. These are all very smart people and they are also acting in self-defence: trying to protect their research fiefdoms in uncertain times. But often I wonder: what monsters have we generated through selection of the fittest! We are cheering people to learn how to absorb money, how to get the best PR to inflate their work, how to become more bombastic and least self-critical. These are our science heroes of the 21st century.

Big Science and Big Pharma have grown ever closer. Astonishingly, most medical researchers do not see this as a conflict of interest, or a threat to their scientific integrity; many of them are irritated that anyone would even bother to question this 'partnership'. Pharmaceutical firms in Britain have increasingly co-located themselves adjacent to prestigious academic medical centres, such as Addenbrooke's Hospital in Cambridge. Large US medical centres like the Cleveland Clinic strongly encourage its medical staff to collaborate with industry. GlaxoSmithKline proudly announced in 2016 that senior biomedical academics would join the 'Immunology Catalyst Sabbatical Programme', 'designed to embed academic scientists in GSK laboratories'. In 2000, Dr Marcia Angell, then editor of the *New England Journal of Medicine* (by common consent the world's most prestigious general medical journal), wrote an editorial entitled 'Is academic medicine for sale?' in which she warned against the increasingly unhealthy relationship between medical researchers and industry, particularly Big Pharma. Shortly after, Dr Thomas J. Ruane wrote to the journal: 'Is academic medicine for sale? No, the current owner is very happy with it.'

The last decade has seen the emergence of a new type of research facility, independent of government and university. These 'cathedral-sized industrial campuses' are funded either by pharmaceutical companies or by billionaire philanthropists such as Eli Broad and Mark Zuckerberg. Zuckerberg and his paediatrician wife, Priscilla Chan, are planning to spend

$3 billion on medical research, with the modest aim to 'cure, prevent or manage all diseases'. (Some commentators have pointed out that $3 billion is a rather small sum for such an ambition.) These centres are beginning to dominate the hugely profitable biotechnology sector. A typical product of such a campus is Novartis's genetically engineered CAR (chimeric antigen receptor) T-cell therapy for childhood acute lymphoblastic leukaemia, which costs $475,000 per patient. The science writer Jim Kozubek has warned that this new biotech is a malign force, widening the gap between rich and poor:

> Biotech, rapidly becoming ever more sophisticated, may be the most powerful cultural force the world has known – and it looks increasingly unfair. Forms of eugenics, *in vitro* fertilization, and the transformations of our very genes and cells into profitable biologic medicines for *investor-first* culture are already being normalized, and inequalities are therefore accelerating. Indeed, the 'artificial world' of biotech, rather than an equitable cultivating force in society that promotes access to medicines and health for the poor and disenfranchised, is enhancing the wealth of elite scientists and their lawyers, while making medicine far more expensive and harder to afford.

'Philanthrocapitalism' – the funding of medical research by the likes of Zuckerberg, Broad and Bill Gates – is a powerful new force in global health. The Bill and Melinda Gates Foundation has done much good, but some have argued that such organizations lack accountability, and that they are used as a shield to deflect criticism of the industries (Microsoft, Facebook) that generated their wealth. Philanthrocapitalism is not new: Rockefeller, Ford and Carnegie cited their charitable activities when responding to criticism of their business methods and treatment of employees. Some new plutocrats, such as the radical libertarian and Trump supporter Peter Thiel, the founder of PayPal, are funding Big Science in the hope that it can buy them the one thing their billions currently cannot: immortality. Many see such philanthrocapitalism as a malign influence on both health care and medical research. The AIDS activist Gregg Gonsalves expressed concern about the Gates Foundation: 'Depending on what side of bed Gates gets out of in the morning, it can shift the terrain of global health... it's not a democracy. It's not even a constitutional monarchy. It's about what Bill and Melinda want.' The Foundation is keen on partnership with pharmaceutical corporations, employing numerous former industry executives. A study published in the *Lancet* in 2009 showed that most of the Foundation's grants went to commercial organizations, and most of the grants to NGOs went to those in high-income countries. David McCoy, Professor of Global Public Health at Queen Mary University London, says: 'Appealing to the megarich to be more charitable is not a solution to global health problems. We need a system that does not create so many billionaires and, until we do that, this kind of philanthropy is either a distraction or potentially harmful to the need for systemic change to the political economy.'

The Human Genome Project (fully completed in 2003) was thought to be the greatest breakthrough of Big Science. James Watson, co-discoverer of the DNA double helix, described it as 'the ultimate tool for understanding ourselves at the molecular level... we used to think our fate was in our stars. Now we know, in large measure, our fate is in our genes.' There were, in fact, two rival genome projects: one was carried out by an international public consortium led by the US and headed by Francis Collins, and the other by Celera, a biotechnology company led by the maverick entrepreneur Craig Venter. In 1999, Collins wrote in the *New England Journal of Medicine* that 'the idea captured the public imagination... in the manner of the great expeditions – those of Lewis and Clark, Sir Edmund Hillary, and even Neil Armstrong.' The completion of a 'rough draft' of the genome was announced on 26 June 2000 at the White House by Bill Clinton, who was joined by Tony Blair on a satellite link. Clinton and Blair declared that all genome information should be free. Collins and Venter announced that the two rival genome projects would co-operate. Clinton, with his great talent for telling people what they want to hear, declared: 'Without a doubt, this is the most important, most wondrous map ever produced by mankind... Today, we are learning the language in which God created life', and confidently predicted that the Human Genome Project would 'revolutionize the diagnosis, prevention and treatment of most, if not all, human diseases'. Blair – who had always struggled with science and technology – piously agreed: 'Today's developments are almost too awesome fully to comprehend.' Francis Collins was slightly overcome by the occasion: 'It's a happy day for the world. It is humbling for me and awe-inspiring to realize that we have caught the first glimpse of our own instruction book, previously known only to God. What a profound responsibility it is to do this work. Historians will consider this a turning point.' In an article published in the *Journal of the American Medical Association* in February 2001, Collins predicted that by 2020, 'new gene-based "designer drugs" will be introduced to the market for diabetes mellitus, hypertension, mental illness, and many other conditions… every tumour will have a precise molecular fingerprint determined, cataloguing the genes that have gone awry, and therapy will be individually targeted to that fingerprint.' Although the print and broadcast media reported uncritically these hyperbolic claims, there were a few dissenters within the academy. Neil Holtzman of Johns Hopkins Medical School and Theresa Marteau of King's College London wrote in the *New England Journal of Medicine* shortly after the White House ceremony:

Differences in social structure, lifestyle, and environment account for much larger proportions of disease than genetic differences. Although we do not contend that the genetic mantle is as imperceptible as the emperor's new clothes were, it is not made of the silks and ermines that some claim it to be. Those who make medical and science policies in the next decade would do well to see beyond the hype.

In 2010, some years after the hype had evaporated, Monika Gisler, from the Swiss science university ETH Zurich, wrote a paper in which she characterized the Human Genome Project as an example of a 'social bubble': 'The hypes fuelling the bubble during its growth have not been followed by real tangible outcomes... the consensus of the scientific community is that it will take decades to exploit the fruits of the HGP [Human Genome Project].'

Collins's predictions have not come to pass. Practical applications of the HGP have been modest, a great disappointment to those who heralded this as the great scientific achievement of *any* age. The psychiatrist Joel Paris observed that when we are told answers are around the corner, that is where they tend to stay. Some of the most eminent figures of American molecular medicine have come clean. The renowned cancer biologist Robert Weinberg admitted that the clinical applications of the Human Genome Project 'have been modest – *very* modest compared to the resources invested'. Harold Varmus, former director of the National Institutes of Health and doyen of American cancer research, wrote in the *New England Journal of Medicine* that 'only a handful of major changes... have entered routine medical practice', and most of them the result of discoveries that preceded the completion of the Human Genome Project. 'Genomics', he said, 'is a way to do science, not medicine.' In 2009, Francis Collins, along with twenty-six other geneticists, wrote a review paper for *Nature*, in which they acknowledged that despite all the effort and money spent, geneticists had not found more than a fractional basis for the common human diseases. 'It is fair to say', Collins admitted, 'that the Human Genome Project has not yet directly affected the health care of most individuals.' Craig Venter, too, confessed: 'There is still some way to go before this capability can have a significant effect on medicine and health.'

Although it failed to deliver the breakthroughs predicted of it, the Human Genome Project has been one of the main drivers of the new age of 'Big Data'. David Pye, scientific director of the Kidscan Children's Cancer Research Charity, warns:

the quantity of data available to researchers is fast becoming a problem. Over the next few years, the computing resources needed to store all the genomic data will be mind boggling (almost 40 exabytes) – far exceeding the requirements of YouTube (one to two exabytes per year) and Twitter (0.02 exabytes per year). Finding the nugget of information that is vital to the production of an effective cure in this mountain of information is looking ever less likely. [An exabyte is 10^{18}, or one quintillion, bytes.]

The failure of Big Science was predicted by the Australian virologist and Nobel Laureate Sir Macfarlane Burnet (1899–1985). His book *Genes, Dreams and Realities* was a sensation when it appeared in 1971. He argued that 'the contribution of laboratory science has virtually come to an end... almost none of modern basic research in the medical sciences has any direct bearing on the prevention of disease or on the improvement of medical care'. Burnet believed that the challenges of the future would not be infectious diseases, but the diseases of civilization, degeneration and old age, and that these would not be conquered like the infectious diseases were during the golden age. Many were outraged by his book, but his eminence ensured that he was taken seriously. His fellow Nobel Laureate, the immunologist Sir Peter Medawar, described *Genes, Dreams and Realities* as an 'extraordinary *lapsus mentis*'. In the *New York Review of Books* in 1980, he wrote: 'As an antidote to Burnet's spiritless declaration I roundly declare that within the next ten years remedies will be found for multiple sclerosis, juvenile diabetes, and at least two forms of cancer at present considered somewhat intractable.' History sided with Burnet, not Medawar, none of whose bold predictions and round declarations came to pass.

The decadence of contemporary biomedical science has a historical parallel in the medieval pre-Reformation papacy. Both began with high ideals. Both were taken over by careerists who corrupted these ideals, while simultaneously paying lip service to them. Both saw the trappings of worldly success as more important than the original ideal. Both created a self-serving high priesthood. The agenda for the profession is set by an academic elite (the hierarchy of bishops and cardinals), while the day-to-day work is done by low-status GPs and hospital doctors (curates, monks). This elite, despite having little to do with actual patient care, is immensely powerful in the appointment of the low-status doctors. Orthodoxy is, in part, established by consensus conferences (church councils). The elite is self-serving, and recruits to its ranks people with similar values and beliefs. The elite is respected by laypeople and has the ear of politicians and princes. The elite collects research funding from laypeople and governments (tithes). This elite is rarely, if ever, challenged, claiming that its authority comes from a higher power (God/Science).

John Ioannidis argues that society at large should lower its expectations: 'Science is a noble endeavour, but it's also a low-yield endeavour. I'm not sure that more than a very small percentage of medical research is ever likely to lead to major improvements in clinical outcomes and quality of life. We should be very comfortable with that fact.' Real science is so hard that it can only be done by a small minority of people who combine high intelligence, passionate curiosity and a commitment to truth. Real science cannot be planned and carried out by committees of bureaucrats and careerists. Contemporary biomedical research has become a danger to both society and medicine. It is a danger because it is scientifically corrupt, and because it serves its own needs, not those of society. Research that has no function other than the production of data and the advancement of careers is self-evidently dangerous. Big Science, for all its boosterism, has been a crushing disappointment. It was inevitably so; most of the major discoveries had already been made during the golden age.

5

THE MEDICAL
MISINFORMATION MESS

In 1948, Francis Avery Jones (then just Dr, not yet *Sir* Francis) recruited a young doctor called Richard Doll to work with him at the Central Middlesex Hospital. Doll joined the hospital's newly established Statistical Research Unit, and worked initially on peptic ulcer disease, showing that Jones's bland diet (milky tea, bramble jelly, sponge cake) was of no benefit. Doll later remarked: 'I have often thought that perhaps that was my most important contribution to gastroenterology, and certainly to public welfare: namely that it was quite unnecessary to have a bland diet if you had a peptic ulcer.' I wonder how Sir Francis reacted to the news that his sponge cake and bramble jelly diet – although doubtless appetizing – was clinically futile? Sir Austin Bradford Hill (1897–1991), professor of medical statistics and epidemiology at the London

School of Hygiene and Tropical Medicine, advised Doll on the statistical design of these ulcer trials. Hill was part of the group convened by the Medical Research Council which conducted the first ever randomized controlled trial in human subjects. It showed 'the clearest possible proof that tuberculosis could be halted by streptomycin'. Hill had set out the principles of clinical-trial design in a series of articles published in the *Lancet* in 1937. These principles are adhered to still, and the streptomycin trial was one of triumphs of postwar British medicine – and the model for all such trials in the future. Hill had a personal stake in the trial: he had served as a pilot during the First World War and was invalided out when he developed chest tuberculosis. He spent two years in hospital and had to abandon his ambition to study medicine; he instead took a degree in economics from the University of London by correspondence. When he had recovered, he went to work with the medical statistician Major Greenwood. Hill was a wise and witty man, and cheerfully admitted to the limitations of medical statistics; he liked to poke fun 'at that most sacred cow, the prospective double blind randomised controlled trial'. He told the story of a conversation with a patient recruited to such a trial: 'Doctor, why did you change my pills?' asked the patient. 'What makes you think that I have?' replied the doctor. 'Well, last week when I threw them down the loo they floated, this week they sink.'

In the late 1940s, Doll turned his attention to cigarette smoking and lung cancer, and worked on this with Hill. It is hard to comprehend now, but at that time, smoking was not regarded as dangerous to health, and more than 80 per cent of the adult male population were smokers. Doll and Jones had earlier investigated the effects of smoking on peptic ulcers, but couldn't reach a definite conclusion because, whether they had a peptic ulcer or didn't, nearly all men smoked; there simply weren't enough non-smokers to make a valid comparison. In a paper published in the *British Medical Journal* in 1950, Doll and Hill showed that smokers had a much higher risk of lung cancer, and the more they smoked, the higher the risk. Association, of course, does not always mean causation, so they followed this with a prospective study of smoking habits and death from lung cancer in doctors. They collected data from doctors on their smoking habits, and followed them up over the next three years to determine how many developed lung cancer, and if so, whether or not they were smokers. This study proved beyond all reasonable doubt that smoking causes lung cancer. Doll's demonstration has saved millions of lives, and he is regarded by many as the greatest medical researcher never to have won the Nobel Prize.

After the war, one of Austin Bradford Hill's students on the diploma course in Public Health at the London School of Hygiene and Tropical Medicine was a young Scot called Archie Cochrane. Brilliant, charismatic and stylish, Cochrane had taken a first in Natural Sciences at Cambridge, studied psychoanalysis in Vienna, and worked in a field ambulance unit during the Spanish Civil War. As a prisoner of the

Germans during the Second World War, he had conducted a randomized controlled trial on yeast as a treatment for the fluid retention common in malnourished prisoners. Inspired by Hill, Cochrane embarked on a career as an epidemiologist, making major contributions to the understanding of lung disease in miners (pneumoconiosis). Cochrane wrote a short book in 1972 called *Effectiveness and Efficiency: Random Reflections on Health Services*, which became an unexpected bestseller. In this book, he argued that the NHS should take evidence from randomized controlled trials to identify which medical treatments worked. Cochrane believed that only treatments of proven effectiveness should be offered by the NHS, and that all such treatments should be costed and delivered equitably.

The rigorous statistical analysis pioneered by Richard Doll, Archie Cochrane and Austin Bradford Hill formed the intellectual and scientific basis for evidence-based medicine, which became the new orthodoxy in the 1990s; it was welcomed by many as a breath of fresh air. The *New York Times* declared evidence-based medicine 'the idea of the year' in 2001, and the phrase 'evidence-based' is now applied to such disparate activities as social science, public policy and even politics. The ideas behind evidence-based medicine were not new. Decades before the term was coined, Richard Asher – who was friendly with both Richard Doll and Archie Cochrane – championed the concept, even if he didn't use this phrase. In his 1961 essay 'Apriority', Asher defined the expression a priori as 'the arguments, reasoning, speculations, notions, traditions, or other support for conclusions which have not been backed by any kind of practical experiment'. From this, he derived his term 'apriority' to describe a kind of lazy thinking, particularly the notion of treatments that have a theoretical reason for why they *might* work, but for which there was no evidence that they *did* work: 'Many things which in theory ought to be highly effective turn out in practice to be completely useless.'

The evidence-based medicine movement began when a group of young, sceptical doctors began to question the received wisdoms of the time – what they disdainfully called 'expert-based medicine'. Brian Haynes, a professor of clinical epidemiology and biostatistics at McMaster University in Hamilton, Ontario (the spiritual home of evidence-based medicine), cited a lecture on Freud at medical school in the late 1960s as his Damascene moment. He asked the lecturer whether there was any evidence that Freud's theories were true. The lecturer replied honestly that there was no such evidence: 'I had an intense tingle in my body as I wondered how much of my medical education was based on unproved theories.' David Sackett – also of McMaster University – is widely regarded as the 'father' of evidence-based medicine. In the late 1960s, he helped establish a new kind of medical school at McMaster, where students studied medicine by starting with a specific patient problem, such as breathlessness, and then learning the relevant anatomy, physiology, pharmacology, and so on. This 'problem-based learning' was combined with statistics and epidemiology, and has become a widely copied model of medical education. Sackett later wrote a bestselling textbook on critical appraisal of research called *Clinical Epidemiology: A Basic Science for Clinical Medicine.* Yet another doctor at McMaster, Gordon Guyatt, coined the phrase 'evidence-based medicine' in 1991 to reflect their internal medicine residency programme, which trained doctors to manage patients on the basis of what the evidence showed worked, not on what the authorities told them to do. Sackett moved to Oxford in 1994, where he became director of the Centre for Evidence-Based Medicine. Unusually for a medical academic, he visited many British district general hospitals, and always began by doing a 'post-take' ward round of the patients admitted the night before with the junior on-call doctors. Sackett showed them how evidence could be useful at the clinical coalface: 'The young physicians realized that they could challenge their seniors in a way that was not possible with expert-based medicine. It was liberating and democratizing.' The epidemiologist Iain Chalmers, along with the obstetrician Murray Enkin, created a database of perinatal trials, which formed the basis for their landmark book *Effective Care in Pregnancy and Childbirth* (1989). This book led to the abandonment of many dangerous practices in obstetrics and neonatology. In 1993, Chalmers established the Cochrane Centre (named in honour of Archie Cochrane). The centre conducts systematic reviews of medical interventions and diagnostic tests; these reviews are published in the Cochrane Library. The Cochrane Centre has 30,000 volunteer experts. I am proud to have been one of them.

Evidence-based medicine (EBM) took off, according to David Sackett, for two reasons: it was supported by senior doctors who were secure enough to be challenged, and it empowered young doctors. A 1996 editorial in the *British Medical Journal* written by Sackett and others successfully rebutted the objections to evidence-based medicine: namely, that it was old hat, impossible to practise, cookbook medicine, the creature of managers and purchasers, and concerned only with randomized trials. EBM was defined by Sackett as 'integrating individual clinical expertise and the best external evidence'. Who could argue with such common sense? EBM introduced the concept of a hierarchy of evidence: at the top was the meta-analysis, or systematic review, which gathers data from all the trials on a given treatment. Below this was the randomized controlled trial (RCT), the gold standard for studies of new drugs. At the bottom of the evidence hierarchy were uncontrolled trials, anecdotal reports and expert opinion. Although its founders would not admit to it, there was nothing new or magical about all this; the new orthodoxy gathered together long-established ideas about sound statistical design, the elimination of logical errors in clinical trials and, most importantly, scientific integrity.

The Cardiac Arrhythmia Suppression Trial (CAST) which began in 1987, was an early triumph for the new approach.

The trial was designed to determine whether drugs that prevented abnormal heart rhythms (antiarrhythmics) reduced mortality after a myocardial infarction (heart attack). Sudden death after a heart attack is often caused by such rhythm disturbances, so it seemed plausible that these drugs might reduce deaths. The trial showed that these drugs did not prevent sudden death: they actually *increased* mortality. It was reckoned – using the alarmist statistics so beloved of evidence-based medicine researchers – that these drugs killed more people every year than were killed during the entire Vietnam War. The routine use of these drugs was a classic example of Richard Asher's 'apriority', and a blow to the mechanistic reasoning that had dominated medicine; by 'mechanistic' I mean the use of a therapy that seems biologically plausible, but for which there is no evidence of benefit. This trial undermined the authority of experts who had up to that point strongly recommended these antiarrhythmic drugs. The drugs may have reduced arrhythmias, but that was a meaningless surrogate metric compared to the prevention of sudden death, an outcome that was hence called 'patient-oriented evidence that matters' (POEMs).

Evidence-based medicine introduced easily understandable statistical concepts, notably 'number needed to treat' (NNT). This is a simple way of communicating the effectiveness of a medical treatment, usually a drug. The NNT is the average number of patients who need to take a drug to prevent one bad outcome, such as a heart attack or a stroke.

A good example is a study published in the *New England Journal of Medicine* in 1998, which examined the benefit of the cholesterol-lowering drug pravastatin (one of a family of drugs known as 'statins') in patients with known coronary heart disease: this is called 'secondary prevention'. The researchers randomized over 9,000 patients to either pravastatin or placebo, and followed them up for 6 years. They reported an impressive-sounding 24 per cent relative reduction in risk of death from heart disease in the group taking the statin compared to the group taking the placebo: 'Over a period of 6.1 years, we estimate that 30 deaths, 28 non-fatal myocardial infarctions, and 9 strokes were avoided in 48 patients for every 1,000 randomly assigned to treatment with pravastatin.' Translating this into 'number needed to treat', it sounds far less exciting: 21 patients need to take the drug for 6 years to prevent an 'adverse event' in 1 patient; 20 of the 21 will not benefit in any way. In studies of statins in 'primary prevention' – where the subjects do not have heart disease – the NNT is in the hundreds. In the West of Scotland Coronary Prevention Study (1995), men aged between 55 and 65, with a serum cholesterol of greater than 6.5 mmol/litre were randomized to pravastatin or placebo for 5 years. The study reported a 28 per cent reduction in deaths from heart disease, but the raw figures tell a different story: 'Treating 1,000 middle-aged men... with pravastatin for 5 years will result in 20 fewer nonfatal myocardial infarctions, 7 fewer deaths from cardiovascular causes, and 2 fewer deaths from other causes': 111 men need to take this drug for 5 years to prevent 1 death; 110 of these men will not benefit. 'Number needed to treat' is much easier to explain to patients than relative and absolute risk, and clearly shows also that most patients taking preventive drugs such as statins and antihypertensives (for high blood pressure) will not gain from years or even decades of taking these drugs, and are far more likely to experience side effects than avoid death from a heart attack. Real patients, however, are seldom told these facts before being prescribed these drugs.

Evidence, unfortunately, is very expensive to produce, mainly because clinical trials are so costly that only Big Pharma companies can afford to run them. Some drug trials are indeed paid for by government-funded agencies such as the Medical Research Council, but these constitute a minority. Three-quarters of trials published in four of the major general medical journals (*Annals of Internal Medicine*, the *Lancet*, the *New England Journal of Medicine* and *JAMA*) are industry funded. If Big Pharma is paying for the evidence, it is hardly surprising if the evidence it produces shows its product in the best possible light; these trials are deliberately designed to maximize the commercial possibilities of the drug. The journals benefit greatly, too: for example, Merck Pharmaceuticals ordered one million reprints of its VIGOR study in 2000 (on the safety of its anti-inflammatory drug Vioxx) from the *New England Journal of Medicine*; these reprints were given to doctors as 'educational' material, enriching the journal by several hundred thousand dollars. Evidence-based medicine, which started as a noble, almost evangelical crusade, is now largely a construct of the pharmaceutical industry. In his book *The Philosophy of Evidence-based Medicine*, Jeremy Howick makes the point that pharma's annexation of EBM does not necessarily invalidate its methodology:

> Imagine for the sake of argument that the EBM philosophy was violently rejected in favour of the view that palm reading experts possessed the unassailable authority to decide whether an intervention had its putative effects. Special interests would then presumably focus on influencing palm reading experts, which could turn out to be far cheaper than conducting several large randomized trials. In brief, the problem that special interests corrupt medical research is a real problem independent of methodology.

Medical research is now so sick that it has itself become a patient, and the object of critical study. The meta-researcher John Ioannidis trained as an epidemiologist during the golden age of evidence-based medicine in the 1990s, working at Harvard, Tufts, Johns Hopkins University and the National Institutes of Health (NIH). As a teenager in Athens, he had achieved some national celebrity as a mathematics prodigy, and these talents proved very useful when he began to critically appraise contemporary medical research. The closer he looked, the more shocked he became: every bit of the process was riddled with error and logical fallacy. Most clinical trials asked the wrong question, recruited too few patients (and those they recruited were often atypical and unrepresentative), analysed the data incorrectly and came to the wrong conclusions. In 2005, Ioannidis published a paper in the journal *PLoS* (*Public Library of Science*) *Medicine*, an online journal whose guiding principle is to publish research which is methodologically sound, regardless of its perceived importance. The paper was provocatively entitled: 'Why most published research findings are false'. This is the summary of the paper:

> a research finding is less likely to be true when the studies conducted in a field are smaller; when effect sizes are smaller; when there is a greater number and lesser preselection of tested relationships; where there is greater flexibility in designs, definitions, outcomes, and analytical modes; when there is greater financial and other interest and prejudice; and when more teams are involved in a scientific field in chase of statistical significance. Simulations show that for most study designs and settings, it is more likely for a research claim to be false than true.

The paper is the most cited and downloaded ever published by *PLoS Medicine*. Astonishingly, most medical researchers privately agreed with Ioannidis: he had simply articulated, in a highly technical, statistical way, what everybody knew. The statistician Douglas Altman (author of the famous *BMJ* paper 'The scandal of poor medical research') said: 'You can question some of the details of John's calculations, but it is hard to argue that the essential ideas aren't absolutely correct.'

Ioannidis then published an analysis of the forty-nine most highly cited research papers in medicine over the previous thirteen years. Forty-five of the forty-nine papers described new treatments. Thirty-four of these studies were repeated, and in fourteen (41 per cent) the original claim was shown to be wrong or grossly exaggerated. Ioannidis turned his attention next to 'nutritional epidemiology', and its vast output of publications linking dietary factors with cancer. Ioannidis and his colleague Jonathan Schoenfeld selected 50 common ingredients from random recipes in *The Boston Cooking-School Cook Book*, and found that 40 (80 per cent) were the subject of 264 studies published in medical journals on their cancer risk: 'Thirty-nine per cent of studies concluded that the studied ingredient conferred an increased risk of malignancy; 33 per cent concluded that there was a decreased risk, 5 per cent concluded that there was a borderline statistically significant effect, and 23 per cent concluded that there was no evidence of a clearly increased or decreased risk.' When Schoenfeld and Ioannidis dissected these studies, they found that 'the great majority of these claims were based on weak statistical evidence', and almost none of these alleged associations was found to be significant when subjected to meta-analysis. Ioannidis told the *Washington Post*: 'I was constantly amazed at how often claims about associations of specific foods with cancer were made, so I wanted to examine systematically the phenomenon. I suspected that most of this literature must be wrong. What we see is that almost everything is claimed to be associated with cancer, and a large portion of these claims seem to be wrong indeed.'

Ioannidis concluded – more in sorrow than in anger – in a 2016 paper for the *Journal of Clinical Epidemiology* that 'evidence-based medicine has been hijacked'. The paper takes the unusual form of a personal letter to his mentor, David Sackett, who had died in 2015:

> The industry runs a large share of the most influential randomized trials. They do them very well… It is just that they often ask the wrong questions with the wrong short-term surrogate outcomes, the wrong analysis, the wrong criteria for success and the wrong inferences…
>
> … corporations should not be asked to practically perform the assessments of their own products. If they are forced to do this, I can't blame them, if they buy the best advertisement (i.e. 'evidence') for whatever they sell.

Sackett, however, was well aware of this hijacking and had written a spoof article many years earlier in 2003 for the *British Medical Journal*, in which he announced the foundation of HARLOT plc that specialized in How to Achieve positive Results without actually Lying to Overcome the Truth:

> HARLOT plc will provide a comprehensive package of services to discriminating trial sponsors who don't want to risk the acceptance and application of their products and policies amid the uncertainties of dispassionate science. Through a series of blind, wholly owned subsidiaries, we can guarantee positive results for the manufacturers of dodgy drugs and devices who are seeking to increase their market shares, for health professional guilds who want to increase the demand for their unnecessary diagnostic and therapeutic services, and for local and national health departments who are seeking to implement irrational and self-serving health policies.

Ioannidis uses the term 'The Medical Misinformation Mess' to encompass all of these issues. Most doctors, and nearly all patients, are unaware of this mess. Even those doctors who are aware generally lack the critical skills needed to evaluate the evidence; they are statistically illiterate. Paul Glasziou, professor of evidence-based medicine at Bond University, Australia, has argued that teaching such critical appraisal skills should be a core part of medical education: 'A twenty-first-century clinician who cannot critically read a study is as unprepared as one who cannot take a blood pressure or examine the cardiovascular system.' Medical education, however, does not encourage scepticism. The Czech polymath and contrarian Petr Skrabanek (1940–94) taught these skills at Trinity College Dublin Medical School during the 1980s and early 1990s, and lamented that 'my course on the critical appraisal of evidence for medical students can be compared to a course on miracles by a Humean sceptic for prospective priests in a theological seminary'. Medical education over-values training and rote memorization at the expense of education, scholarship and the cultivation of the critical faculty.

The most important thing I learned during the three years I spent as a research fellow is that nearly all papers in medical journals are dross. Ioannidis, along with other meta-researchers such as Glasziou and Sir Iain Chalmers, estimate that about 85 per cent of medical research is useless and wasted. This global waste amounts to £170 billion annually. As far back as 1954, Richard Asher warned that 'the danger of crooked statistics is that its fallacies are less likely to be noticed because of the mixture of awe, suspicion, and reverence with which statistical thinking is regarded by most of us'. Alvan Feinstein warned about excessive reliance on randomized controlled trials and meta-analyses in 1997, and predicted the advent of authoritarian practice guidelines:

The laudable goal of making clinical decisions based on evidence can be impaired by the restricted quality and scope of what is collected as 'best available evidence'.

The authoritative aura given to the collection, however, may lead to major abuses that produce inappropriate guidelines or doctrinaire dogmas for clinical practice.

Evidence-based medicine, Feinstein argued, did not reflect the demographic shift towards older, frailer patients with several chronic diseases (comorbidities), taking as its evidence data from trials on younger patients with single diseases. Such evidence oversimplified the many complex variables of the clinical encounter, and the goals that are important to real people. Feinstein attacked, too, the fascination with meta-analysis, which he called 'statistical alchemy for the twenty-first century'. Many others have criticized meta-analysis, arguing that researchers combine different types of studies – they are comparing apples and oranges; that they often exclude 'negative' studies; and that they often include low-quality studies ('garbage in, garbage out'). Meta-analysis, however, remains the least worst tool we have.

Alvan Feinstein's prediction that evidence-based medicine would lead to prescriptive guidelines came true, with massive over-prescribing, particularly in the elderly. The 2004 NHS contract for GPs heavily incentivized preventive prescribing (for high blood pressure, cholesterol, osteoporosis), contributing to a huge increase in the volume of medication consumed by the British population. Twenty per cent of all adults in Scotland are on five or more long-term medications. In the US, 25 per cent of people in their sixties arc on five or more medications, rising to 46 per cent of people in their seventies, and 91 per cent of nursing-home residents. Feinstein also correctly pointed out that the evidence supporting the use of these drugs was based on studies of younger, healthier people, not the kind of patients who ended up taking them. The oldest, sickest people – nursing-home residents – are generally excluded from trials of new drugs, yet they are the most medicated people in our society. Sick and dying people are commonly sent in from nursing homes to the kind of acute general hospital where I work. Most are on ten or more medications, which are continued even when the person has clearly entered the terminal stage of their lives: the average survival of a person entering a nursing home in Ireland is two years. These patients are also far more likely to experience side effects and drug interactions, and to die of these 'adverse reactions'.

Over-prescribing ('polypharmacy') is now such a major public health issue – particularly in the elderly – that it has, somewhat ironically, become the subject of a new field of research. My brother Denis, an academic geriatrician, has devoted his career to it. Polypharmacy is the direct cause of major side effects and increased mortality, and a huge waste of money. The people most likely to experience side effects of prescribed drugs are those over eighty, with multiple comorbidities and a life expectancy of three years or less. One prescription often leads to another: a drug given for high blood pressure may cause ankle swelling due to fluid retention, leading to another prescription for a diuretic (water tablet), which may cause potassium depletion, leading to a prescription for potassium tablets, which may cause nausea, leading to a prescription for antiemetic drugs, which may cause confusion, and on, and on, a process known as the prescribing cascade. Fifteen per cent of acute admissions to hospital in elderly people are due to drug side effects.

Taken individually, the prescribing of each drug can be justified on the basis of available evidence: yes, a statin lowers the *risk* of a heart attack or stroke; yes, a drug to lower blood pressure lowers the *risk* of stroke; yes, aspirin lowers the *risk* of a heart attack; yes, this drug for osteoporosis lowers the *risk* of a fracture; yes, an anticoagulant lowers the *risk* of stroke, and on, and on. What evidence-based medicine doesn't tell us is whether the *combination* of all these drugs, in this specific, individual, unique person, is beneficial or harmful. Statins – taken for high cholesterol – are one of the great triumphs of Pharma. High cholesterol is only one of many factors associated with heart disease, which include smoking, high blood pressure, diabetes and family history. Once started on a statin, the 'patient' continues to take it for the rest of their life. As we have seen, the vast majority of people taking statins every day do not benefit, yet people with advanced dementia and other 'life-limiting' conditions commonly take statins to lower the risk of a heart attack or stroke in their non-existent future. We are treating populations, not people. The cholesterol awareness campaign has been so successful that very elderly people, and patients with other diseases that will carry them off long before their heart gives out, commonly ask me to check their cholesterol levels. It can be difficult to explain that cholesterol is only one of many risk factors, and that medication to lower it will probably do them no good and might even cause harm. The drug companies know well that the medical outpatients clinic or the GP surgery is not the environment which facilitates these nuanced discussions of benefit and risk. It's so much easier to write a prescription for a statin. Before the patent expired, Lipitor – a statin – was the biggest-selling drug in the world. Between 1996 and 2012, Lipitor made $125 billion for Pfizer. Meanwhile, in poor countries, millions of people die every year in unnecessary pain because they have no access to morphine.

GPs are often blamed for this over-prescribing, but there is a cultural expectation – particularly in Ireland and Britain – that a visit to the doctor must conclude with the issuing of a prescription. Doctors also find this gesture a useful means of concluding a prolonged and demanding consultation; a polite way, as one GP put it, of saying 'now fuck off'. Drugs are commonly prescribed for people with relatively mild, transient depression and anxiety because doctors do not have the time or resources to offer psychological therapies. Both patients and doctors over-estimate the benefits of drugs, and under-estimate their risks. I commonly see patients – usually from nursing homes – who are taking up to twenty prescribed medications. Deprescribing is much more difficult than prescribing, involving, as it does, lengthy discussions on balancing risks and benefits, discussions that many people are either not able to have or unwilling to have. Older patients may view such deprescribing as a sign that their doctor is giving up on them, while some doctors regard deprescribing as a criticism of the colleague who first prescribed the medication. My brother has developed criteria to detect inappropriate pre-scribing: for example, giving a patient two drugs which are known to adversely interact with each other. I am more con-cerned, however, about 'appropriate' prescribing: that which, although sanctioned by 'evidence' and enforced by guidelines and protocols, is unlikely to benefit the individual patient.

Kieran Sweeney (1952–2009) was a GP and academic who questioned the philosophical basis of evidence-based medi-cine. He pointed out – as did many others – that this evidence comes from studies of populations, and

the results relate to what happens in groups of people, rather than in an individual. Decisions are based on interpretation of the evidence by objective criteria, dis-tant from the patient and the consultation. Subjective evidence is anathema. In this context, evidence-based medicine is almost always doctor-centred; it focuses on the doctor's objective interpretation of the evidence, and diminishes the importance of human relationships and the role of the other partner in the consultation – the patient.

Sweeney argued that there is a 'personal significance', beyond statistical significance and clinical significance: what matters most to this person now? The role of the doctor, he argued, is to evaluate the available evidence, explore the patient's aspirations and preferences, and advise accordingly. The doctor's experience, training and personality will influence this discussion, but 'the patient's contribution is more important'.

Medicine is an applied, not a pure science. Many would say that it is not a science at all: it is a craft, a practice. Even the phrase 'scientific medicine' implies that we don't really believe that medicine is a science. After all, does anyone use the phrase 'scientific physics'? In many ways, science and medicine are antithetical: doubt is at the very core of science, but doctors who express doubt are not highly regarded by their patients. This reflects the contemporary combination of consumerism in health care and the Cartesian belief that our bodies are machines, and should be mended as efficiently and unfussily as a broken kitchen appliance. The most successful doctors are those who make a clear and unambiguous diagnosis, and who give the patient complete faith in the treatment. This is why complementary and alternative medicine remains so popular. Its practitioners are always absolutely definite as to the cause of their patients' problems; depending on which church the practitioner belongs to, this could be allergy to yeast, or misaligned vertebrae. It doesn't matter. What counts is the absolute certainty with which this diagnosis is conveyed.

Belief in the efficacy of the treatment is similarly instilled. Most of the problems that prompt people to visit doctors are transient and self-limiting; they get better regardless of what is done. This explains the continuing success of complementary medicine: nature heals, and the homeopath gets the fee and the credit. They are occasionally found out when they take on more serious problems, particularly cancer.

There is a paradox at the heart of medicine: its intellectual basis is scientific in its ethos, but practice is not. The rational scepticism of David Hume is the basis of scientific thinking, but is a positive handicap for the doctor who, unlike Richard Doll, Petr Skrabanek, Austin Bradford Hill, Archie Cochrane, Thomas McKeown and John Ioannidis, sees real patients. We deal with people, with all of their irrationality, variation, vulnerability and gullibility. Science informs medicine, and medicine looks to science for answers, but they are radically different, often opposing, activities. Although eminent and pompous doctors like to quote the philosopher of science Karl Popper, the Popperian scientist, with ideas of bold conjecture and merciless refutation, does not flourish in medicine. There is little or no evidence to support quite a lot of what we do, and doctors have to work within, and around, this limitation. A project called 'Clinical Evidence', sponsored by the *British Medical Journal*, reviewed 3,000 medical practices, including treatments and tests. They found that a third are effective, 15 per cent are harmful, and 50 per cent are of unknown effectiveness. Medicine adopts new practices quickly, but drops them slowly. Over the last twenty-five years there have been some evidence-based medicine successes, in areas such as surgery and endoscopy, which are outside the baleful influence of pharma. Many useless, once routine procedures have been abandoned. Most doctors, however, work in a world where managing uncertainty is the greatest skill, and most patients have trivial, self-limiting conditions, or chronic shit life syndrome. Hospital-based general medicine is mainly concerned with the management of frail old people with multiple problems – medical, social and existential. A 'post-take' general medical ward round seems a long way from the Popperian idea of science.

Richard Asher, who somehow managed to be both a Humean sceptic and a clinical doctor, observed that whatever the evidence says, success in medical practice is often due to a combination of real enthusiasm on the part of the doctor and blind faith in the patient. He argued that you cannot fake such enthusiasm: 'If you admit to yourself that the treatment you are giving is frankly inactive, you will inspire little confidence in your patients, unless you happen to be a remarkably gifted actor, and the results of your treatment will be negligible.' Asher's paradox – 'a little credulity makes us better doctors, though worse research workers' – is why medicine is so difficult for the Humean sceptic. When I was a very young and inexperienced house officer, a wise rheumatologist, whose outpatients I assisted with, told me: 'You will find this clinic much easier if you can bring yourself to believe in the concept of soft-tissue rheumatism.' ('Soft-tissue rheumatism' is a blanket term used to describe all manner of muscle and joint aches – often psychosomatic – which cannot be given a definite diagnosis by X-rays or blood tests.) The Spanish philosopher and essayist José Ortega y Gasset in his *Mission of the University* (1930) expressed this well: 'Medicine is not a science but a profession, a matter of practice… It goes to science and takes whatever results of research it considers efficacious; but it leaves all the rest. It leaves particularly what is most characteristic of science: the cultivation of the problematic and doubtful.'

The founders of evidence-based medicine did not foresee the sins that would be committed in its name. When clinical guidelines first appeared in the 1990s, I welcomed them as a useful educational tool. Gradually, however, guidelines became mandatory protocols. These protocols, we were told, were all 'evidence-based', but many would not withstand for very long the beady gaze of John Ioannidis. In the US, protocols were driven by the insurance companies, and in Britain by the NHS, supported by a vast number of professional bodies and quangos. Although protocols are supposedly evidence-based, there is little evidence that their adoption and implementation has led to any significant improvements. Some believe that protocol-driven care is a prelude to a future when most medical care is provided by paraprofessionals, such as physician assistants and nurse practitioners.

The Israeli behavioural psychologists Daniel Kahneman and Amos Tversky persuaded the world that humans are inherently flawed, their reasoning subject to systematic cognitive bias and error. The idea of an individual doctor exercising clinical judgement, using unquantifiable attributes such as experience and intuition, has become unfashionable and discredited, yet it is this judgement, this human touch, which is the heart of medicine. Richard Asher defined 'common sense' as 'the capacity to see the obvious even amid confusion, and to do the obviously right thing rather than working to rule, or by dead reckoning'. The most powerful therapy at doctors' disposal is themselves.

6

HOW TO INVENT A DISEASE

The medical–industrial complex has undermined the integrity of evidence-based medicine. It has also subverted nosology (the classification of diseases) by the invention of pseudo-diseases to create new markets. A couple of years ago, I stumbled across a new pseudo-disease: 'non-coeliac gluten sensitivity'. I was invited to give a talk at a conference for food scientists on gluten-free foods. I guessed that I was not their first choice. Although I had published several papers on coeliac disease during my research fellowship, I had written only sporadically on the subject since then; I was not regarded as a 'key opinion leader' in the field. I was asked to specifically address whether gluten sensitivity might be a contributory factor in irritable bowel syndrome (IBS). This is a common, often stress-related condition that causes a variety of symptoms, such as abdominal pain, bloating and diarrhoea. It is probably the most frequent diagnosis made at my outpatient clinic.

Coeliac disease is known to be caused by a reaction to gluten in genetically predisposed people, but now many others, who despite having negative tests (biopsy, blood antibodies) for coeliac disease, still *believe* their trouble is caused by gluten. This phenomenon has been given the label of 'non-coeliac gluten sensitivity'. At the conference, an Italian doctor spoke enthusiastically about this new entity, which she claimed was very common and responsible for a variety of maladies, including IBS and chronic fatigue. I told the food scientists that I found little evidence that gluten sensitivity had any role in IBS, or indeed anything other than coeliac disease. I listened to several other talks, and was rather surprised that the main thrust of these lectures was commercial. A director from Bord Bia (the Irish Food Board) talked about the booming market in 'free-from' foods: not just gluten free, but lactose free, nut free, soya free, and so on. A marketing expert from the local University Business School gave advice on how to sell these products – he even used the word 'semiotics' when describing the packaging of gluten-free foods. Non-coeliac gluten sensitivity may not be real, but many people at this conference clearly had invested in its existence. One speaker showed a slide documenting the exponential rise in journal publications on gluten sensitivity, and it reminded me of Wim Dicke, who made the single greatest discovery in coeliac disease – that the disease was caused by gluten – and struggled to get his work published.

Willem-Karel Dicke (1905–62) was a paediatrician who practised at the Juliana Children's Hospital in The Hague, and later (after the Second World War) at the Wilhelmina Children's Hospital in Utrecht. He looked after many children with coeliac disease. This was then a mysterious condition which caused malabsorption of nutrients in food, leading to diarrhoea, weight loss, anaemia and growth failure. Many had bone deformity due to rickets (caused by lack of vitamin D), and death was not uncommon: a 1939 paper by Christopher Hardwick of Great Ormond Street Children's Hospital in London reported a mortality rate of 30 per cent among coeliac children. Hardwick described how these children died: 'The diarrhoea was increased, dehydration became intense, and the final picture was that of death from a severe enteritis.' It had long been suspected that the disease was food-related, and various diets, such as Dr Haas's banana diet, were tried, but none was consistently effective. During the 1930s, Dicke had heard of several anecdotal cases of coeliac children who improved when wheat was excluded from their diet. Towards the end of the Second World War, during the winter of 1944–5 – the *hongerwinter*, or 'winter of starvation' – Holland experienced a severe shortage of many foods, including bread, and the Dutch were famously reduced to eating tulip bulbs. Dicke noticed that his coeliac children appeared to be getting better when their 'gruel' was made from rice or potato flour instead of the usual wheat. He attended the International Congress of Pediatrics in New York in 1947, and although he was a shy and reticent man, he told as many of his colleagues as he could about his observation on wheat and coeliac disease. Years later, Dicke's colleague and collaborator, the biochemist Jan van de Kamer, wrote: 'Nobody believed him and he came back from the States very disappointed but unshocked in his opinion.'

Dicke moved to Utrecht, and formed a research partnership with van de Kamer, who had developed a method for measuring the fat content of faeces. This was a means of quantifying the malabsorption of food from the intestine in these children: the greater the stool fat content, the greater the malabsorption. He began a series of clinical trials of wheat exclusion, and showed that coeliac children got better on this diet. By measuring faecal fat content before and after wheat exclusion, he produced objective evidence of the benefit of this diet. Later, he showed that gluten (the protein which gives bread its elastic quality) was the component in wheat responsible for the disease. Dicke wrote a paper describing his findings and sent it to one of the main American paediatric journals. He did not receive even an acknowledgement, and the manuscript wasn't sent out for review. Meanwhile, a research group at Birmingham University and the Birmingham Children's Hospital had heard of Dicke's work and wanted to test his findings. One of that group, Charlotte Anderson, visited Dicke to see his studies of coeliac children at first hand. He went out of his way to help Anderson with her research; she later paid tribute to 'his old-world gentility'. Dicke had formally written up his work for his doctoral thesis, presented to the University of Utrecht in 1950. He also sent off a paper to another journal – the Swedish publication *Acta Paediatrica Scandinavica*. This paper was accepted, but by the time it eventually appeared in print, the *Lancet* had published a paper by the Birmingham group confirming Dicke's findings. Dicke died young, at fifty-seven, after a series of strokes.

When I began my research on coeliac disease in the 1980s, it was a well-recognized, although relatively uncommon, condition: about 1 in every 2,000 people in Britain were diagnosed with it. It was then much more prevalent in Ireland, particularly in Co. Galway, where the disease was diagnosed in 1 in every 300. In retrospect, this was at least partly due to the fact that the professors of medicine and paediatrics at University College Galway at that time both had a special interest in the condition and actively sought it out. Making a formal diagnosis of coeliac disease in the 1980s was difficult, requiring the prolonged and distressing Crosby capsule intestinal biopsy. (The patient had to swallow a steel bullet – the capsule – attached to a hollow tubing, and wait for at least two hours for the capsule to reach the small intestine.) Gradually, however, the diagnosis became easier. By the late 1980s, biopsies could be obtained using an endoscope, in a procedure that took five or ten minutes; in the 1990s, blood antibody tests became widely available, and were shown to be highly accurate. The ease of these diagnostic tests, along with greater awareness of the condition, led to a steep rise in diagnosis of coeliac disease during the 1990s and 2000s: about 1 per cent of the British and Irish population are now thought to have coeliac disease, although many – possibly most – remain undiagnosed. Coeliac disease is no longer regarded as primarily a disease of children: the diagnosis can be made at any age. Several screening studies (using blood antibody tests) across Europe and the US show that the prevalence of coeliac disease is somewhere between 1 and 2 per cent of the population. The treatment – a gluten-free diet – is lifelong and effective.

The patients I diagnosed with coeliac disease in the 1980s were often very sick. Nowadays, most adults diagnosed with the condition have minimal or no symptoms. The ease of diagnosis and increased public awareness led many people with various chronic undiagnosed ailments to seek tests for coeliac disease. These 'medically unexplained' conditions included IBS, chronic fatigue and fibromyalgia. A few did indeed have coeliac disease, but most didn't. Undaunted by negative tests for coeliac disease, some – encouraged by stories in the media – tried a gluten-free diet, and felt better. Their doctors attributed this to suggestibility and the placebo effect. Many complementary and alternative medicine practitioners, however, thought it was a real phenomenon, and began to recommend a gluten-free diet for all sorts of chronic ailments. These patients were not satisfied with reassurances along the lines of 'well, you're not coeliac but if it makes you feel better, give the diet a go', and demanded a formal diagnostic label for what ailed them. As the bitter history of chronic fatigue syndrome/ME has shown, patients with 'medically unexplained' symptoms are often resistant to psychological formulations. Our contemporary culture, for all its superficial familiarity with psychology and its vocabulary, remains uncomfortable with the notion of 'psychosomatic' disease. Many of my IBS patients prefer gluten sensitivity to 'stress' as the explanation for their symptoms, just as some people with chronic fatigue believe they have an infection with the bacterium that causes Lyme disease. Doctors now spend much of their time manoeuvring the ever-widening gap between their patients' beliefs and their own.

By the new millennium, coeliac disease researchers had run out of new ideas: the disease was easily diagnosed and easily treated – what was left to know? Then along came a new opportunity called non-coeliac gluten sensitivity. In February 2011, fifteen coeliac disease researchers from around the world met at a hotel near Heathrow Airport. They were keen to give this phenomenon of self-diagnosed gluten sensitivity some form of medical credibility, or, as they put it, to 'develop a consensus on new nomenclature and classification of gluten-related disorders'. They were not shy about the commercial agenda: 'The number of individuals embracing a gluten-free diet appears much higher than the projected number of coeliac disease patients, fuelling a global market of gluten-free products approaching $2.5 billion in global sales in 2010.' The meeting was sponsored by Dr Schär, a leading manufacturer of gluten-free foods. A summary of this meeting was published in the journal *BMC Medicine* in 2012. Non-coeliac gluten sensitivity now became an officially recognized part of 'the spectrum of gluten-related disorders'. Dr Schär must have been pleased with this consensus, which led to several studies on non-coeliac gluten sensitivity over the next few years. Most of these studies were poorly designed, badly written up, and published in low-impact, minor journals, the sort of work that John Ioannidis would eviscerate with relish. One of the very few well-designed studies, from Monash University in Melbourne, published in the prestigious US journal *Gastro-enterology*, found that people with self-reported gluten sensitivity did not react to gluten (disguised in pellets) any more than they did to a placebo.

Despite these inconclusive studies, many review articles appeared in the medical journals describing the symptoms of non-coeliac gluten sensitivity and how to diagnose it. Several of these papers appeared in the journal *Nutrients*, which, for a period, featured in a list of predatory journals. Professor Carlo Catassi, an Italian paediatrician, has published several papers on non-coeliac gluten sensitivity, mainly in *Nutrients*. He is probably the most prominent name associated with the condition and has received 'consultancy funding' from the

Dr Schär Institute. In a 2015 review article for the *Annals of Nutrition and Metabolism*, Catassi listed the following as clinical manifestations of non-coeliac gluten sensitivity: bloating, abdominal pain, lack of wellbeing, tiredness, diarrhoea, nausea, aerophagia (swallowing air), gastro-oesophageal reflux, mouth ulcers, constipation, headache, anxiety, 'foggy mind', numbness, joint and muscle pain, skin rash, weight loss, anaemia, loss of balance, depression, rhinitis, asthma, weight gain, cystitis, irregular periods, 'sensory' symptoms, disturbed sleep pattern, hallucinations, mood swings, autism, schizophrenia, and finally – my favourite – ingrown hairs. In a Disclosure Statement, we are told that 'the writing of this article was supported by Nestlé Nutrition Institute'.

Professor Catassi is the first author, too, of a paper entitled 'Diagnosis of non-coeliac gluten sensitivity (NCGS): the Salerno Experts criteria', also published in *Nutrients.* In October 2014, a group of thirty 'international experts' met in Salerno, Italy, 'to reach a consensus on how the diagnosis of non-coeliac gluten sensitivity should be confirmed'. The meeting was again funded by Dr Schär. Only six of the fifteen experts who met at Heathrow in 2011 made it to Salerno: was there a schism in the church of gluten sensitivity? The experts gave us criteria to diagnose a condition that probably doesn't exist. Non-coeliac gluten sensitivity is thus a model for what might be called a post-modern disease. It does not have a validated biological marker (such as a blood test or a biopsy), and the diagnosis is made on the basis of a dubious and highly arbitrary symptom score. Its 'discovery' owes much to patient pressure and the suborning of expert opinion by commercial interests. I found a picture online of the experts gathered at Salerno, and was reminded of a fresco in the Sistine Chapel depicting the first Council of Nicea in AD 325. The council was convened by the emperor Constantine to establish doctrinal orthodoxy within the early Christian Church. The industry-sponsored get-together in Salerno had similar aims. Why did these experts attach their names to a consensus on how to diagnose this pseudo-disease? Unlike Willem-Karel Dicke, a clinical doctor who stumbled on an idea he desperately wanted to test, the Salerno experts are typical contemporary biomedical researchers: their motivation is professional, rather than scientific. Few share Dicke's qualities of modesty, reticence and 'old-world gentility'. Their aim is expansionist: the establishment of a new disease by consensus statement, the Big Science equivalent of a papal bull. Non-coeliac gluten sensitivity has been decreed by this edict, just as papal infallibility was decreed by the First Vatican Council in 1870. The creation of this new disease benefits the researchers, who now claim many more millions of 'patients'; it benefits the food industry, with dramatic rises in sales of 'free-from' foods; and it benefits people with psychosomatic complaints, who can now claim the more socially acceptable diagnosis of non-coeliac gluten sensitivity. If so many people are benefiting from all of this, why worry about science, or truth?

Consensus statements have been part of the medical academic landscape since the 1970s, and frequently mocked as GOBSAT ('good old boys sat around a table'). The American Psychiatric Association decided in 1973 that homosexuality was no longer a disease: this depathologization was declared by consensus, after a vote among the association's members. Although it is unlikely, they could just as easily redeclare it as a disease. Petr Skrabanek wrote on the phenomenon of consensus conferences in 1990:

> the very need for consensus stems from lack of consensus. Why make an issue of agreeing on something that everyone (or nearly everyone) takes for granted? In science, lack of consensus does not bring about the urge to hammer out a consensus by assembling participants whose dogmatic views are well known and who welcome an opportunity to have them reinforced by mutual backslapping. On the contrary, scientists are provided with a strong impetus to go back to the benches and do more experiments.

Consensus conferences very often facilitate the aims in particular of pharma, by expanding the pool of 'patients' who might need their product. Consensus statements, for example, set the levels above which cholesterol levels and blood pressure is 'abnormal' and must be 'treated'. Careful selection of participants guarantees the 'right' consensus. In the 'hierarchy of evidence' espoused by evidence-based medicine, however, consensus statements are near the bottom, slightly above 'a bloke told me down the pub'. 'The consensus of experts', remarked Alvan Feinstein, 'has been a traditional source of all the errors that have been established through-out medical history.' The British mathematician Raymond Lyttleton coined the term 'the Gold Effect' (after his friend, the Austrian physicist Thomas Gold) in 1979. In *Follies and Fallacies in Medicine* (1989), James McCormick and Petr Skrabanek explained how the Gold Effect transforms belief in some idea into certainty: 'Articles on the idea, initially starting with "Evidence has accumulated", rapidly move to articles that open "The generally accepted", and before long to "It is well established", and finally to "It is self-evident that".'

Although the coeliac disease experts accepted commercial sponsorship and then obligingly legitimized the highly dubious entity that is non-coeliac gluten sensitivity, two entrepreneurial American doctors, William Davis, author of *Wheat Belly* (2011), and David Perlmutter, author of *Grain Brain* (2013), took the public awareness of gluten to the next level. Their bestselling books contributed substantially to the popular perception of gluten as toxic not just for coeliacs, but for *everyone*. Davis (a cardiologist) argues that 'modern' wheat is a 'perfect, chronic poison', that it is addictive and is the main cause of the current obesity epidemic. Perlmutter (a neurologist) claims that 'modern grains are destroying your brain', causing not only Alzheimer's disease, but also 'chronic headaches, depression, epilepsy and extreme moodiness'. This is, of course, absurd, and completely unsupported by any evidence, but it is a model of restraint compared to Professor Catassi's list of 'clinical manifestations of gluten sensitivity'. Perlmutter's and Davis's books have sold in their hundreds of thousands, but are dismissed by scientists. Science, however, should be more concerned about the reputational damage inflicted on it by the feverish musings of the Salerno experts.

All of this has created a whole new market, with new consumers. YouGov, the UK-based market-research firm, produced a report in 2015 called 'Understanding the FreeFrom consumer'. Gluten-free is not the only 'free-from' food: consumers can choose lactose free, dairy free, nut free, soya free and many other products. Ten per cent of the UK population are 'cutting down' on gluten; remarkably, two-thirds of those cutting down on gluten do not have a sensitivity, self-diagnosed or otherwise, and are referred to as 'lifestylers' by the marketing experts. Lifestylers tend to be young, of high social class, female, vegetarian, regular exercisers, and 'spiritual but not religious'. The 'free-from' food market in Britain is booming, with annual sales of £740 million; gluten-free products make up 59 per cent of it. This market is growing at a rate of roughly 30 per cent annually. Twenty million Americans claim that they experienced symptoms after eating gluten. One-third of adults in the US say they are reducing or eliminating their gluten intake. You can buy gluten-free shampoo and even go on a gluten-free holiday.

It is easy to mock this foolishness, and many do: look up J. P. Sears's 'How to become gluten intolerant' on YouTube. Meanwhile, several celebrities, including Gwyneth Paltrow, Miley Cyrus and Novak Djokovic, have proclaimed the benefits of gluten avoidance. 'Everyone should try no gluten for a week!' tweeted Miley Cyrus. 'The change in your skin, physical and mental health is amazing! U won't go back!' The gluten-free food market, which had hitherto been a small, niche business, has expanded rapidly over the last several years. In 2014, sales of gluten-free foods in the US totalled $12.18 billion; it has been estimated that the market will grow to $23.9 billion by 2020.

With the exception of the 1 per cent of the population who are coeliac, there is no evidence that gluten is harmful. There is, however, growing evidence that a gluten-free diet in non-coeliac people may carry a risk of heart disease, because such a diet reduces the intake of whole grains, which protect against cardiovascular disease. Fred Brouns, professor of health food innovation management at Maastricht University, wrote the pithily entitled review 'Does wheat make us fat and sick?' for the *Journal of Cereal Science* in 2013. He examined the claims made against wheat by both William Davis and David Perlmutter – namely, that it causes weight gain, makes us diabetic and is addictive. He addressed also the charge (made by Davis, Perlmutter *and* the Heathrow experts) that modern wheat contains higher levels of 'toxic' proteins. Brouns and his colleagues reviewed all the available scientific literature on wheat biochemistry, and concluded that wheat (particularly whole wheat) has significant health benefits, including reduced rates of type 2 diabetes and heart disease. He found no evidence that the wheat we eat now is in any way different from that consumed during the Palaeolithic era, apart from having higher yields and being more resistant to pests. Genetically modified wheat has not been marketed or grown commercially in any country. 'There is no evidence', he concluded, 'that selective breeding has resulted in detrimental effects on the nutritional properties or health benefits of the wheat grain.'

Alan Levinovitz, a professor of religion at James Madison University in Virginia, was struck by the parallels between contemporary American fears about gluten and the story of the 'grain-free' monks of ancient China. These early Daoists, who flourished 2,000 years ago, believed that the 'five grains' (which included millet, hemp and rice) were 'the scissors that cut off life', and led to disease and death. The monks believed that a diet free of the five grains led to perfect health, immortality and even the ability to fly. In his book *The Gluten Lie* Levinovitz places contemporary American anxieties about gluten in a long line of food-related myths: 'As with MSG, the public's expectation of harm from gluten is fuelled by highly profitable, unscientific fearmongering, validated by credentialed doctors. These doctors tap into deep-rooted worries about modernity and technology, identify a single cause of all our problems, and offer an easy solution.'

Does it really matter if many people adhere to a gluten-free diet unnecessarily? After all, it's their own choice, and if they're happy with it, why should we bread eaters fret? The gluten story is a symptom of the growing gap between rich and poor. For most of human history, the main anxiety about food was the lack of it. Now, the worried well regard food as full of threats to their health and are willing to pay a premium for 'free-from' products. People who do not have scientific knowledge are likely to take the food industry's claims at face value, and their children, bombarded with advertising on social media and television, will add to the pressure. When food was scarce, fussiness about it was frowned upon and socially stigmatized because it was wasteful of a precious resource. What used to be simple fussiness has now progressed to self-righteous grandstanding, and self-diagnosed food intolerance is often the first step on the *via dolorosa* of a chronic eating disorder.

We have a strange paradox: the majority of people who *should* be on a gluten-free diet (those with coeliac disease) aren't, because most people with coeliac disease remain undiagnosed. The majority of those who *are* on a gluten-free diet shouldn't be, because they do not have coeliac disease. The 'lifestylers' are deluded, and non-coeliac gluten sensitivity is a pseudo-disease. People with coeliac disease are ambivalent about the gluten-free fad: they have benefited, because gluten-free produce is now easily obtained, and restaurants and supermarkets are very gluten aware. They resent, however, the narcissistic lifestylers and the self-diagnosed gluten intolerant for trivializing the condition of the 1 per cent who really do need to go gluten free.

The Great Discovery in coeliac disease was made by Wim Dicke. This was a typical breakthrough from medicine's golden age, achieved by a determined clinical doctor who worked with little financial or institutional support. Although Dicke struggled to publish his crucial discovery, since then thousands and thousands of papers have been published on coeliac disease, many – like mine – describing immunological epiphenomena of no clinical significance or benefit to patients. John Platt's observation that most research studies produce bricks that 'just lie around in the brickyard' sums up most of coeliac disease research; I am ashamed to admit that I produced a few of these bricks. Coeliac disease is easily diagnosed and easily treated, yet the coeliac research cavalcade trundles on, with its conferences and consensus statements. Dicke is a fine example of the amateur researcher from the golden age. His integrity and reticence, not to mention his willingness to assist other researchers, now seem quaint. His inspiration during the *hongerwinter* saved the lives of many sick children. I wonder what this humble old-fashioned doctor would have made of non-coeliac gluten sensitivity, the Salerno experts, and Miley Cyrus.

7

'STOP THE AWARENESS NOW'

'Despite the uncertainty with regard to diagnosis and pathophysiology,' wrote Anna Krigel and Benjamin Lebwohl from Columbia University, 'public awareness of NCGS [non-coeliac gluten sensitivity] is growing.' The gluten-sensitivity researchers often cite this 'awareness' as a justification for their activities. Awareness raising is a ploy dear to the medical–industrial complex. Every week, I receive free copies of two medical newspapers. Many of the pages are filled with photographs of hospital consultants at conferences, or GPs at golf outings wearing garish sportswear. A new genre of staged photograph has emerged over the past few years: the Raising Awareness picture. The object of this awareness raising could be any of the diseases, common or rare, that afflict us. The group shown to be aiming the spotlight of publicity at this disease is usually a combination of the following: a nervous-looking doctor who is an expert in that disease; a proud patient; a representative from the pharmaceutical company that produces a drug for that disease; the chief executive of the association which represents patients with the disease; and the joker – a politician, a media celebrity or a sportsperson. The group is usually posed along with some sort of encouraging slogan. Each member of the group has their own reasons to pose for the camera. The doctor is playing the new game of My Disease Is Better Than Your Disease, hoping that all this hoopla will generate money for research, staff and facilities while raising his or her professional profile. The pharmaceutical company naturally anticipates increased sales for their product. The patient isn't used to media attention, but quite likes it. The chief executive – usually the only full-time employee of the disease association – hopes that this awareness raising will generate enough money to keep him or her in a job. The politician will pose for anything: a retired cabinet minister appears in these free papers almost every other week, raising awareness of all kinds of diseases. The media celebrity or sports star may well have been paid a fee. Everyone has gained.

Patient-support groups usually start out with the best of intentions, but they are invariably and inevitably hijacked by industry and dominated by single-issue extremists. I have some experience of giving talks to these groups, and after some years, declined these invitations. When I worked in the NHS, I regularly attended the annual meeting of a local support group for people with colitis and Crohn's disease. Most of these people were charming and welcoming, but every year I encountered 'the milkman'. I do not know if he was a patient or the relative of a patient, but he sustained, year after year, the delusion that Crohn's disease was spread by the consumption of milk contaminated with *Mycobacterium paratuberculosis* (closely related to the bacterium that causes tuberculosis). Although several studies had conclusively eliminated this bacterium as a possible cause of Crohn's disease, every year 'the milkman' raised his hand during the question-and-answer session to ask why I wasn't lobbying for a complete ban on milk sales.

Disease-awareness campaigns are based on certain assumptions, namely: that if the general public knew more about this disease, they would feel more kindly disposed towards its victims, and might even donate money to the lobby group; that politicians – so attuned to that which is modish – might be more inclined to fund new treatments and facilities for that disease; and that if awareness is insufficiently raised, other diseases will elbow this disease out of the way when it comes to giving money – both charitable donations and government funding. It is a rather dwarfish view of the world and of medicine, but it is largely true. Ireland, a small country with a population of fewer than five million, supports hundreds of disease-specific patient-support groups. Although the charity sector in Ireland has lost some of its lustre following a series of financial scandals, high-profile individuals such as ex-politicians are commonly employed as chief executives of such groups, because their experience of dealing with the media is highly valued. Ireland has one of the worst health services in the European Union; acute hospitals permanently operate at over 100 per cent capacity, and 15 per cent of the entire population are on a waiting list to see a hospital consultant. The Irish electoral system (proportional representation) means that politicians are very vulnerable to local concerns, such as small district general hospitals. Decisions on health care are therefore made very often for political reasons, and the sheer size of the health lobby sector in Ireland reflects this.

A clearly frustrated Joe Harbison, a stroke specialist at St James's Hospital in Dublin, and head of the Irish Health Service's National Stroke Programme, wrote a piece for the *Irish Times* in 2016 entitled 'Stroke patients are no less deserving than cancer patients'. He argued that new, highly expensive cancer drugs were getting funded, while the less glamorous disease of stroke was left languishing: 'The cost to provide one of these [cancer] drugs for a single year is more than has been spent on the national stroke programme since its inception seven years ago.' In a thinly veiled dig at the bellicose Irish 'cancer community', Harbison wrote:

> Our ground-breaking therapies should not be discounted because our patients are less able to advocate for them. Health service spending needs to be prioritised

according to which interventions provide the greatest level of benefit for the resources made available. Deciding priorities by whoever can gain the attention of the media and politicians will eventually create more losers than winners. Those with the least resources for advocacy and those least able to articulate their case will end up with the worst care.

Doctors are willing participants in the raising-awareness game. An oncologist shares little common ground with a stroke physician; they are competitors for limited resources. An honourable conscientious objector to the my-disease-is-better-than-your-disease arms race is the psychiatrist Professor Sir Simon Wessely, former president of the Royal College of Psychiatrists, who told the *British Medical Journal*:

> Every time we have a mental health awareness week my spirits sink. We don't need people to be more aware. We can't deal with the ones who already are aware... We should stop the awareness now. In fact, if anything, we might be getting too aware. One wonders what is happening when you have 78 per cent of students telling their union that they have mental health problems – you have to think, 'Well, this seems unlikely.'

Wessely pointed out that although celebrities such as Prince Harry have tried to publicize and destigmatize mental illness, psychiatry struggles to recruit trainees, and services for physical and mental illness remain almost completely segregated. Despite all the awareness raising, Wessely argues that the medical profession itself is prejudiced against both psychiatry and people with mental illness. A psychiatrist friend told me that people with serious chronic mental illness, such as schizophrenia, are the real losers in all this awareness raising. These patients struggle to access good treatment, both medical and psychiatric, and their life expectancy is significantly lower than the general population. He wryly observed that the politicians who publicly support suicide awareness campaigns and call for the provision of more counsellors, might better redirect their efforts to addressing poverty and unemployment, the main drivers of suicide.

Meanwhile, life's inevitable struggles, vicissitudes and difficulties have been rebranded as psychopathologies, what my friend calls 'the societal intolerance of distress'. Simon Wessely dismissed the charge that the psychiatric profession is part of a global conspiracy to make everyone mentally ill: 'We do the opposite. We really are the people who try to maintain some form of boundary between sadness and depression, between eccentricity and autism, between shyness and social phobia.' Maintaining this boundary is difficult. Hospital-based psychiatrists quite correctly devote their professional energies to treating patients with the most serious and chronic mental illnesses, but GPs, with consultation times of five to ten minutes, can only manage this vast societal intolerance of distress with a prescription for an antidepressant.

As I write, today, 2 April, is World Autism Awareness Day. There are five other health awareness days in April: World Health Day on 7 April; World Homeopathy Day on 10 April; World Haemophilia Day on 17 April; and World Malaria Day on 25 April. In my hospital, I am regularly exposed to these holy days, as the doctors and nurses concerned with the disease which they wish to raise my awareness of set up stalls at the front entrance to the hospital and outside the canteen. On World Diabetes Day (14 November), for example, I can have my blood glucose checked, while on World Hypertension Day (17 May), I can have my blood pressure measured. There are now so many awareness days that we experience 'narcotizing dysfunction', a term coined by the sociologists Paul Lazarsfeld and Robert Merton in 1957 to mean that the more we learn about an issue from the media, the less likely are we to do anything about it. We are bombarded with information about health and disease. Some recent awareness campaigns have taken this gimmickry to absurd levels. The Ice-Bucket Challenge appeared in 2012, intending to raise awareness of motor neurone disease (MND). The craze peaked in 2014, driven by its unique combination of celebrity narcissism, bullying and social media virtue signalling. It all got a little out of hand when Macmillan Cancer Support was accused of hijacking the Ice-Bucket Challenge – sure proof, if one was needed, of the existence of the my-disease-is-better-than-your-disease phenomenon. The Irish prime minister Leo Varadkar is both admired and reviled for his canny use of social media. His website shows him having buckets of icy water poured over him at Trinity College Dublin. Varadkar is soaking wet as the Trinity students douse him, but displays a fixed, good-sport rictus. Sitting on either side of him, also drenched and smiling manically, is the head of the Trinity College Medical School and the CEO of the Irish Health Research Board.

Some disease-awareness campaigns have been so success-ful that they have led to protocol-enforced dramatic changes to the way doctors work, even when the evidence for such protocols is debatable. The most striking example of such a campaign is sepsis. Infection, historically the biggest killer of humans, has been rebranded as 'sepsis'. Sepsis could mean anything from pneumonia in an elderly woman to septi-caemia (blood poisoning) in a twelve-year-old following a scratch. One such twelve-year-old was Rory Staunton, who in 2012 died in New York. He had injured his arm playing basketball, and was unlucky enough to develop septicaemia as a result. He was even more unlucky when both the family paediatrician and the doctors in the emergency room of a New York hospital failed to recognize how ill he was. Bereaved families often channel their grief into awareness-raising campaigns, and Rory's Irish-born father Ciaran, a political lobbyist, set up the Rory Staunton Foundation for Sepsis Prevention. The foundation lobbied successfully for a senate hearing on sepsis, held in 2013. This led to the state of New York adopting regulations that require all hospitals to put in place protocols for screening and treating sepsis. Furthermore, all school children in the state now have mandatory sepsis education.

Rory's Regulations is an example of what might be called 'sentimentality-based medicine'. Bereaved people are regarded as having not only a special moral authority, but a medical one, too. Maurice Saatchi, for example, embarked on a quixotic attempt to bring in new legislation on cancer research after the death of his wife Josephine Hart, and was indulged by many who should have known better. Had Ciaran Staunton not been a professional lobbyist, we would probably never have heard of Rory. He has been given a platform by the medical profession to raise awareness of sepsis, and regularly gives lectures at hospitals, including my own. How could you possibly question a man whose opening statement at medical conferences is: 'My heart is broken'? How could you possibly express doubts about the over-prescribing of antibiotics and inappropriate treatment of frail elderly patients to a man who pauses regularly during lectures to rein in his tears? He has stated that since the adoption of Rory's Regulations, 5,000 lives have been saved in New York State alone. How could you possibly question a man such as this about these dubious statistics? Ciaran Staunton has been indulged because the worst thing that can happen to a parent has happened to him. A cavalcade of sepsis advocates, who saw a professional opportunity for expansion, has emerged. Their mission, they say, is to 'raise awareness' of sepsis; boosters usually have other, less visible agendas. They can be spotted by their use of jumbo jet statistics, frequent media appearances and courting (and rather cynical use) of lay champions like Ciaran Staunton.

Mandatory sepsis protocols now exist in all hospitals. The 'warning triggers' for sepsis are so vague that huge numbers of elderly hospital patients are subjected to the Sepsis Six, which include the administration of intravenous fluids and antibiotics, and the insertion of a urinary catheter. In order to qualify for the Sepsis Six, a patient has to meet only two of the following criteria: heart rate over 90; respiratory (breathing) rate over 20; temperature greater than 38°C, or less than 36°C; altered level of consciousness; blood glucose greater than 7.7; or white cell count greater than 12 or less than 4. A great many sick old people meet these criteria, most of whom don't have sepsis and find themselves on fluids and antibiotics that they don't need, and with a catheter in their bladder. Ciaran Staunton is correct that doctors need to be aware of sepsis, but we also have to be aware of the risks in old people of intravenous fluids (heart failure), antibiotics (*Clostridium difficile* infection) and urinary catheters (sepsis, paradoxically). Doctors have to be aware of a great many things, which is why our selection is so rigorous, and our training so long.

There is growing disquiet about sepsis protocols. A group

from the Harvard Medical School voiced these concerns in the *New England Journal of Medicine* in 2014:

> Sepsis mandates are not without risk… Protocols that force physician behaviour risk promoting inappropriate prescribing of broad-spectrum antibiotics for non-infectious conditions, unnecessary testing, overuse of invasive catheters, diversion of scarce ICU capacity, and delayed identification of non-sepsis diagnoses.

In June 2017, the *New England Journal of Medicine* published a study of more than 49,000 patients treated for sepsis in hospitals in New York State over the first two years (2014–16) after Rory's Regulations were introduced. The study reported that for every hour that doctors failed to initiate the sepsis protocol (the 'three-hour bundle'), mortality rates climbed between 3 and 4 per cent. The Rory Staunton Foundation claimed, on the basis of this study, that the mandatory sepsis protocols had saved over 5,000 lives in New York. Not everyone was convinced. Mervyn Singer, a sepsis expert and professor of intensive care medicine at University College London, pointed out that mortality in the patients who did not complete the treatment protocol within three hours was 23.6 per cent; the rate in those who did complete the protocol within this time was only marginally lower at 22.6 per cent. Singer remarked: 'The idea that every hour makes a difference forces doctors to think they're racing against time. And I'd argue that the three-hour window for some patients makes no difference whatsoever.' The trial was retrospective and non-randomized, and the authors conceded that 'the results may be biased by confounding'. One such confounding factor is the appropriateness of the initial choice of antibiotic, for which no data were available. The claim that this study proved that 5,000 lives were 'saved' by the introduction of Rory's Regulations is absurd. Rory Staunton died of bad luck: not just one oversight, but a series of mistakes – the classic Swiss cheese model of medical error – and not because of a global ignorance of sepsis on the part of the medical profession. Meanwhile, I see many patients misdiagnosed as having sepsis, some of whom are seriously harmed by the sepsis-focused treatment given to them. This is because most people with sepsis aren't twelve-year-old boys who got unlucky after a scratch.

A few months ago, I saw one of the haematology consultants sitting at a desk by the front entrance of my hospital; next to the desk was a poster announcing that today (13 October) was World Thrombosis Day. Some patients admitted to hospital develop a clot in the veins in their calf, called a deep vein thrombosis (DVT); in some cases, these clots dislodge and travel to the lungs, causing a pulmonary embolus (PE), which can be fatal. DVTs and PEs are collectively known as venous thromboembolism (VTE), and the highest risk is in patients undergoing surgery, particularly orthopaedic procedures such as hip replacement. These patients are routinely given an injection with an anticoagulant (blood-thinning) drug called heparin, which significantly reduces the risk of developing such clots. There is consensus that these high-risk patients should be given heparin, but now *all* patients admitted to UK and Irish hospitals must undergo a tick-box assessment of their risk of clotting. Any patient over the age of sixty is regarded as being at risk. As most hospital patients are over sixty, the overwhelming majority of patients admitted acutely are now given heparin. One of the largest meta-analyses of this practice found that heparin decreased the risk of pulmonary embolus, but not DVT, and that there was no reduction in mortality. More worryingly, for every clot prevented, two major bleeds were caused. You need to give heparin to about 400 patients to prevent an embolus in one. This is not exactly persuasive data, yet the great majority of patients admitted to my hospital are given heparin, because a protocol forces the junior admitting doctor to do so. A poster advertising World Thrombosis Day is prominently displayed on my ward; the poster proclaims: 'Everyone has a RIGHT to know if they are at risk of developing VTE.'

Guidelines are just that: they *guide*. Protocols, however, are mandatory. Protocols such as those for suspected sepsis assume that doctors are incapable of recognizing sick patients and treating them in a timely and sensible manner. A sepsis protocol might have saved Rory Staunton; we shall never know. Sepsis protocols have come with a huge cost in terms of over-diagnosis and inappropriate treatment. The medical profession has blandly and bovinely accepted this. Sepsis protocols are driven by intensive care specialists who have a very narrow telescopic view. They see the teenage patient with septicaemia, but they don't have to make a judgement on the eighty-five-year-old lady on the general medical ward who, because she is slightly confused and has a pulse rate greater than 90, has triggered the Sepsis Six, even though she probably doesn't have sepsis. Similarly, haematologists drive the VTE prophylaxis protocols because they see the patients with PEs; they never see the patients who develop a major bleed from the heparin. These various specialists see only their own tiny quarter of the medical swamp. The rest of us are obliged to deal with the messiness and uncertainty.

Pharma's single greatest idea was to move its focus from the sick to the well, thus creating vast new markets of 'patients' requiring a lifetime of treatment with drugs like statins. Ivan Illich predicted this: 'A culture can become the prey of a pharmaceutical invasion. Each culture has its poisons, its remedies, its placebos, and its ritual settings for their administration. Most of these are destined for the healthy rather than the sick.' The medical establishment dismissed Illich as a crank and a 'Jeremiah', yet forty years on, much of what he warned against has come to pass. Illich's prophesy that the pharmaceutical invasion would be aimed at the healthy rather than the sick has indeed come true, with the advent of 'disease mongering': the creation of new markets for drugs by redefining large populations of healthy people as being in need of whatever drug is being marketed. This is where awareness campaigns really come into their own. Having been encouraged by patient groups and doctors to get tested or screened, large numbers of people who hitherto thought of themselves as healthy, find that they are at risk of developing some disease in the future because of their blood pressure or cholesterol levels. They are told that a particular medication will lower that risk, and that they will need to take this medication for the rest of their lives. Disease mongering, wrote Iona Heath, has 'meant a shift of attention from the sick to the well and from the poor to the rich'.

To achieve this vast expansion, pharma needed the co-operation of the medical profession, particularly medical academics, who are known in the trade as 'key opinion leaders'. The company typically sets up an advisory board stuffed with such handsomely paid 'leaders'. This board advises the company on how best to shape professional opinion, usually though pseudo-educational meetings, sponsored supplements given out with medical journals and the establishment of new guidelines. The patient-support groups are wooed with money and educational material. Although pharmaceutical companies are banned in Ireland from advertising directly to the public, they get around this by sponsoring awareness campaigns on radio, newspapers, television and social media. Some of these campaigns are so well disguised that they are almost undetectable. I came across an article recently in the

Irish Times with the emotive title 'Patient organisations shouldn't have to march on the streets to get access to medicines'. The author Sylvia Thompson wrote: 'The Irish Platform for Patient Organizations, Science and Industry (IPPOSI) has expressed concern that new, innovative and improved drugs will not be available or will be significantly delayed to patients in Ireland.' IPPOSI, according to its website, 'is a patient-led organization that works with patients, government, industry, science and academia to put patients at the heart of health innovation'. The eighteen board members are a mixture of medical academics, pharmaceutical corporation executives and representatives of disease advocacy groups. It is not clear how this body is funded, but the *Irish Times* article was accompanied by the statement 'Brought to you by the *Irish Times* Content Studio', which according to the paper's website 'has been developed to drive brand stories, engage audiences with commercial content and to enhance the working relationship with our many commercial partners'.

Drug companies argue that they meet a demand, that they operate in a market, just like any other commercial enterprise. This is not really true, because the market is gamed; demand is artificially created and then inflated. Medical academics are suborned, or even bribed, to talk up the new product. These inducements typically include lucrative invitations to speak at 'satellite' sessions at medical conferences. Conference delegates are attracted to these symposia with free food and drink. These events were traditionally regarded as separate from the conference, but over the last several years, they have begun to appear in the main programme. I attended one such industry-sponsored event at the British Society of Gastro-enterology some years ago; the company concerned wanted to raise awareness of its very expensive drug for colitis and Crohn's disease. The symposium was chaired by a famous television newsreader, not a recognized medical leader in the field of inflammatory bowel disease. He bore an expression of perplexity throughout the proceedings, as if he had wandered into the wrong room, and struggled both with the scientific terminology and the names of the panel members.

The drug companies commonly fund patient-support groups; these support groups are bombarded with boosterist information about new drugs, which they then lobby for, as is commonly the case with cancer drugs. The relevant medical academics often give lectures to the support groups extolling the new drug, which in turn boosts the demand. The ease with which the medical profession has been recruited for these campaigns is remarkable. Academic doctors sometimes plead financial need; membership of an advisory board often covers the school fees. 'It's very rewarding', one professor archly informed me. And lest I be accused of pompous and self-righteous grandstanding, I can confess that I have accepted my share of pharma's bounty. I justified this to myself with the usual lame excuse that everybody else was doing it; it took me a long time to locate my conscience. In the late 1990s, I attended a session at a conference where two speakers debated whether a new biological drug was a 'magic bullet' for a particular intestinal disease. At the end of the debate, a show of hands was taken of the audience, who, by a large majority, voted that this drug was most definitely *not* a magic bullet. I was surprised, therefore, when some months later, I received a glossy newsletter, purporting to be an educational supplement, which carried an article on the conference debate I had attended. The author reported that a large majority of the attendees had agreed that this drug truly *was* a magic bullet. I had few illusions about how pharma worked, but this was astonishing. I wrote a formal letter of complaint to the Association of the British Pharmaceutical Industry. They upheld my complaint, and issued the company concerned with a small fine. Shortly after, one of the company's managers approached me at a conference, wondering if my wife and I would like to attend an educational meeting in Florida. I declined – the first step on my road to conversion to No Free Lunch Fundamentalism.

The creation of these vast new markets has enriched pharma so much that global revenues in 2014 were more than $1 trillion. Meanwhile, the sick languish. The population are subjected to more and more screening programmes (for breast cancer, cervical cancer, colon cancer, high blood pressure, cholesterol levels, etc., etc.), but if they become acutely ill and need to go to hospital, it is likely that they will spend hours on a trolley in an emergency department. When they are finally admitted to a ward, it is often chaotic, squalid and understaffed. Hospices have to rely on charity just to keep going, and have so few beds that ten times as many people die in general hospitals than hospices.

Medicine should surely prioritize the sick, the dying and the vulnerable. Decisions on how money is spent on health care should be based on need not on sentimentality, and certainly not on the basis of lobbying by special-interest, disease-specific patient groups. So put your ice bucket away. Cancel the photo shoot. Disband your patient-support group. Stop pestering the healthy with awareness campaigns. Lobby, if you must, for humane treatment of frail, old people in emergency departments, but let's not raise awareness.

8

THE NEVER-ENDING
WAR ON CANCER

In the hierarchy of awareness raising, cancer is king. In 1971, Richard Nixon signed the National Cancer Act, promising to make 'the conquest of cancer a crusade'. Nixon had a keen sense for what exercised his fellow Americans, and surmised that cancer had replaced nuclear annihilation as their greatest fear. He never used the phrase 'War on Cancer', but it is as indelibly linked to his name as the word 'Watergate'. Nixon predicted that the National Cancer Act would prove to be the most significant achievement of his administration. The most bellicose of the new crusaders predicted that cancer would be 'licked' in time for the bicentennial celebrations in 1976. This optimism, in some ways, was not unreasonable. Hadn't America put a man on the moon only two years before? The decades since the Second World War had seen remarkable progress in medicine: infectious disease had been largely conquered – why not cancer? But Nixon didn't defeat cancer, which is now overtaking heart disease as the number one killer of Americans. In the forty-odd years from 1971 to 2012, $500 billion was spent on cancer research – $20,000 for every American who has died of cancer. There have been many modest – and a few spectacular – advances in cancer treatment since 1971, but for many of the common cancers, such as lung and pancreas, there has been little or no improvement in survival since Nixon signed the Cancer Act. The billions invested in elucidating the cell biology and genetic mutations has resulted in precious little of practical use. The monolithic and narrow scope of Big Science is to blame, as it devotes most of its efforts towards mechanistic 'explication' – documenting the biology of cancer cells – and little to 'intervention' or actual treatment. The cancer researcher David Pye put it succinctly: 'How can we know so much about the causes and progression of disease, yet do so little to prevent death and incapacity?' Cancer is a disease (or group of diseases) mainly of old age: if we lived long enough, we would all eventually get it. As the number of old people is steadily increasing, cancer keeps outrunning us.

Cancer research is big business and has many stakeholders and beneficiaries. Barack Obama and Joe Biden launched their 'Cancer Moonshot' in 2016. Biden said: 'I'm going to devote the rest of my life to working on this, and I think we're perilously close to making some gigantic progress.' Obama went even further: 'Let's make America the country that cures cancer once and for all.' Even the vocabulary around cancer ('moonshot') is infected with a sort of hubristic oedema, a malignant hypertrophy. We live in a culture that focuses almost exclusively on benefit, and rarely considers cost. Progress in curing cancer is now reminiscent of the trench combat of the First World War, where a few hundred yards of territory might be gained at the expense of thousands of dead. Each new meagre, incremental advance is hailed as a 'breakthrough' or a 'game changer'.

The pharmaceutical companies who produce new cancer drugs, and the oncologists who carry out clinical trials on them, routinely use meaningless surrogate endpoints in these trials, such as 'disease-free remission' and 'reduction in tumour size', instead of traditional hard outcomes, such as survival. Two Canadian oncologists, Christopher Booth and Elizabeth Eisenhauer of the National Cancer Institute of Canada Clinical Trials Group at Queen's University, Ontario, attacked such bogus statistics in a paper published in the *Journal of Clinical Oncology* in 2012 entitled 'Progression-free survival: meaningful or simply measurable?' Progression-free survival is defined as 'the length of time during and after the treatment of a disease, such as cancer, that a patient lives with the disease but it does not get worse'. In the case of cancer, this means that the tumour is still present, but not increasing in size. The authors describe the increase in the number of randomized controlled trials of new drugs for metastatic cancers using this metric as the primary endpoint:

> Some trials showing improvement in progression-free survival, without a corresponding increase in overall survival, have led to approval of new drugs and/or changes in standard of care. This suggests a growing belief in the oncology community that delaying progression in metastatic disease is a worthy goal, even if overall survival is not improved. But is a new treatment that improves progression-free survival really an advance for patients? Or is it only lowering the bar to declare active some of our much-heralded new molecular targeted therapies? We believe that as a community, this trend requires discussion and debate.

An improvement in progression-free survival for most cancer patients simply means that their cancer is no bigger on the CT scan, but they don't live any longer. Booth and Eisenhauer concluded that progression-free survival was neither clinically significant for doctors, nor existentially meaningful for patients, and cited the use of such bogus metrics as an example of the McNamara, or quantitative, fallacy, which I will discuss later.

Most of these new cancer drugs are very, very expensive. Patients stricken with cancer, not surprisingly, want to access the very latest treatment, regardless of the evidence of benefit

– or lack of it. In Britain, new drugs are assessed by the government agency called the National Institute for Health and Care Excellence (NICE), which uses a number of criteria to determine whether these new agents offer benefit and value for money. (Archie Cochrane had argued for this kind of cost/benefit assessment in 1972.) Many such drugs are turned down by NICE, leading to a predictable public outcry. In response to this protest, the prime minister, David Cameron, set up a special fund to pay for cancer drugs that had either been rejected by NICE or were awaiting assessment. The fund paid out £1.27 billion between 2010 and 2016. In 2017, a group of health services researchers at the London School of Hygiene and Tropical Medicine published an analysis of this spending in the cancer journal *Annals of Oncology*. Of the 47 drugs funded, only 18 (38 per cent) improved survival, and then only by a meagre average of 3 months. The remaining 29 had no benefit, and caused significant side effects. The senior author, Professor Richard Sullivan from the Institute of Cancer Policy at King's College London, told the *Guardian* that the Cancer Drugs Fund had been 'a massive health error'. He went on: 'In science, we demand levels of evidence, but public policy is opinion-based, not evidence-based. You can't have that in health. Populism doesn't work.'

Populism doesn't cure cancer, but it trumps justice, evidence and fairness every time. In 2016, hospices in Britain cost a total of £868 million. The money wasted on the Cancer Drugs Fund would have paid for every hospice in the UK for a year-and-a-half. The medical–industrial complex is a very devious bully, fantastically adept at recruiting the general public: who could possibly be against more spending on cancer? What kind of monster could possibly question giving a dying person a chance, no matter how small? How can you possibly put a price on a human life? Meanwhile, some oncologists stoke the demand: they casually mention a new 'experimental' treatment to the patient and their family. If you're dying of cancer, you'll try anything. Cancer patient-support groups – very often funded by drug companies – lobby for access to the new drugs. In the NHS, there is the phenomenon of 'postcode prescribing', where some health authorities will fund cancer drugs and others will not. Some cancer patients beg, borrow or crowdfund the cost of the last futile throw of the dice.

One such patient was Anthony Wilson, broadcaster, night-club owner and music impresario. He was diagnosed with kidney cancer in 2006. He underwent surgery, but the cancer had spread (metastasized). Standard chemotherapy failed, and his oncologist recommended Sunitinib ('Sutent'), a new drug for metastatic kidney cancer. Wilson's local health authority in Manchester refused to fund this drug, which then cost £3,500 a month. BBC news reported in July 2007 that a group of Wilson's friends had set up a fund to pay for the drug. Wilson said: 'This is my only real option. It is not a cure but can hold the cancer back, so I will probably be on it until I die... I've never paid for private healthcare because I'm a socialist. Now I find you can get tummy tucks and cosmetic surgery on the NHS but not the drugs I need to stay alive. It's a scandal.' One of the largest trials of Sunitinib was carried out by the Memorial Sloan Kettering Cancer Center in New York – one of the great cathedrals of modern oncology – and was published in the *Journal of Clinical Oncology* in 2009. They compared Sunitinib with the standard drug for metastatic kidney cancer, interferon alpha. Sunitinib increased survival by 4 months (26.4 v. 21.8 months), hardly a dramatic improvement. The study, predictably, also measured the usual meaningless surrogate endpoints, such as 'progression-free survival' and 'objective response rate'. Wilson died in August 2007 at the Christie Cancer Hospital in Manchester; his oncologist claimed that his death was unrelated to his cancer.

Drugs and chemotherapy generally do little for patients with advanced cancer. They come with a high cost, both in terms of their price and their side effects, and because the clamour for them from patients and oncologists elbows aside other, better ways of improving cancer survival, such as prevention and earlier diagnosis. A 2004 meta-analysis examined whether chemotherapy drugs improved survival in patients with 'solid' cancers (as opposed to blood cancers, such as leukaemia). Chemotherapy prolonged survival in some, such as testicular cancer, Hodgkin's disease, cancer of the cervix, lymphoma and ovarian cancer. These cancers, however, added up to only 10 per cent of all cases. In the other 90 per cent of cancers (breast, lung, colon, prostate), chemotherapy improved survival by only 3 months. In 2005, a paper in the *British Journal of Cancer* looked at 14 consecutive new cancer drugs approved by the European Medicines Agency, and found the average extra life gained was a miserly 1.2 months. More recently, 48 new drugs approved by the US Food and Drug Administration between 2002 and 2014 gave a median 2.1 month survival benefit.

Many expert commentators have expressed concern about trials of cancer drugs. Peter Wise, a physician and researcher at Charing Cross Hospital in London, waited until after retirement to write a damning analysis of cancer drug trials for the *British Medical Journal* entitled 'Cancer drugs, survival, and ethics':

> Many drugs approved on the basis of better progression-free survival have been subsequently found not to produce better overall survival than the comparator drug. Some of these drugs are logically withdrawn but others remain inexplicably on the market.
>
> Surrogate endpoints [meaningless outcomes such as progression-free survival] are also used by the FDA [the US Food and Drug Administration] and EMA [European Medicine Agency] for accelerated and conditional approval, respectively, of what are judged to be urgently needed new drugs. A 2010 FDA review revealed that 45 per cent of cancer drugs given accelerated approvals were not granted full approval, either because subsequent trials

failed to confirm effectiveness or because the results of trials were not submitted. One reason may be the industry's reluctance to communicate negative results...

The FDA's decision to introduce a 'breakthrough' category in 2012 compounds the risks of premature approval on limited evidence. The pressure for early approval is enhanced by lobbying from patient advocacy groups, prompted by industry and with often premature media announcements of drugs that are 'game changing', 'groundbreaking', 'revolutionary', 'miracle', or other unjustifiable superlatives. The risky practice of approval before proof gains even more momentum.

In the US, the 2016 21st Century Cures Act modified the FDA drug approval process, and lowered even further the evidentiary standards for new drugs; the bill had bipartisan support, pushed by more than 1,400 lobbyists.

The journalist A. A. Gill was diagnosed with metastatic lung cancer in 2016, aged sixty-two. He announced his illness in the *Sunday Times*, where he was a regular contributor as a restaurant critic and TV reviewer: 'In truth, I've got an embarrassment of cancer, the full English. There is barely a morsel of offal not included. I have a trucker's gut-buster, gimpy, malevolent, meaty malignancy.' He wrote about his treatment in his last-ever piece for the *Sunday Times*. At his first meeting with an oncologist at Charing Cross Hospital in London, he asked about chemotherapy:

Well, there's a new treatment, immunotherapy. It's the biggest breakthrough in cancer treatment for decades… It's new and it's still being trialled, but we're a long way along the line and it is the way cancer treatment is bound to go. It's better for some growths than others, but it's particularly successful with yours. If you were in Germany or Scandinavia or Japan or America, or with the right insurance here, this is what you would be treated with.

Gill's partner Nicola Formby asked the oncologist if he would get better treatment as a private (rather than NHS) patient: 'If he had insurance, I'd put him on immunotherapy – specifically nivolumab. As would every oncologist in the First World. But I can't do it on the National Health.' Gill researched the wonder drug: 'The National Institute for Health and Care Excellence (NICE), the quango that acts as the quartermaster for the health service, won't pay. Nivolumab is too expensive – £60,000 to £100,000 a year for a lung-cancer patient; about four times the cost of chemo.' Gill's article appeared in the *Sunday Times Magazine* on 11 December 2016. The end of the piece states: 'Since A. A. Gill wrote this article he has started nivolumab.' The *Sunday Times* didn't mention the other thing Gill did since he had written the article: he died the day before the piece came out, too late, it would appear, for the news to get to the printing presses. I was troubled when I read this article. Gill clearly spent much of the few months between diagnosis and death fretting about the failure of the NHS to treat him with nivolumab. I was even more troubled by the fact that his oncologist dangled before this dying man a drug that he knew he couldn't prescribe.

Drugs like nivolumab, which give very modest survival gains in most, work spectacularly well in the occasional patient. They are like lottery tickets, but are presented to the patient as a sure thing. Six months after A. A. Gill's death, the *New England Journal of Medicine* published a randomized trial comparing nivolumab with the standard platinum-based chemotherapy for stage IV lung cancer. Median survival in the nivolumab group was 14.4 months versus 13.2 months in the chemotherapy group: not exactly a paradigm shift or game changer, or 'the biggest breakthrough in cancer treatment for decades'. In 2015, 46,388 people were diagnosed with lung cancer in Britain. Even if only a quarter of this number qualified for nivolumab, and were treated for a year, the cost would be somewhere between £0.7 billion and £1 billion, roughly what is spent every year on hospice care in Britain. And this is the problem with these debates: the sad story of A. A. Gill is told without context. We assume that all these decisions about paying for new cancer drugs occur in isolation, that there are no consequences for the rest of the health service or society in general. This is sentimentality in its true and pernicious form. The medical–industrial complex relies on this childishness. We claim to respect science and the scientific method, but we don't really understand it, so our decisions on the applications of science are irrational. I have used the example of the under-funding of hospice care, but the real danger of this alleged 'progress' is not to other aspects of health care, but to our society at large. We must have higher, and better, priorities than feeble, incremental and attritional extension of survival in patients with incurable cancer. Some medical–industrial bully (or tabloid journalist) will retort: 'Surely extending A. A Gill's life by even a few months is worth £100,000?' This is always followed by the trump card: 'How can you put a price on a life?' Predictably, NICE recommended, in November 2017, that the Cancer Drugs Fund pay for nivolumab in patients with a particular type of lung cancer (squamous cell) who have already been treated with chemotherapy.

'Precision' medicine refers to the matching of cancer patients with drugs that target the genes driving their disease. Currently, patients with lung and breast cancer are routinely screened for particular genetic mutations, but new-generation genetic sequencing can screen for hundreds of mutations, either in a sample taken from the tumour, or even in a blood test (a 'liquid biopsy'). Many new cancer drugs target a specific gene mutation, rather than a type (lung, breast, colon) of cancer. According to advocates of precision medicine, the genetics of a tumour are more important than its location. This new molecular profiling is currently very expensive, and produces a great deal of data that doctors often don't know how to interpret. Another limitation of this approach is that cancers are very effective at developing resistance to drugs, and developing new mutations. New genomics companies, such as Foundation Medicine, offer a 'portfolio of genomic tests', interrogating more than 300 genes and matching the patient's tumour to the best available current therapies. This company has built up a cancer genomics database called FoundationCore™ from 180,000 patient records, and works 'with more than 30 biopharma partners'. Their mission statement contains the ominous phrase 'We never give up'.

Although genomics and precision medicine have so far not led to any dramatic improvement in cancer survival, we can be sure that this genetics-driven paradigm will drive up the already inflated cost of cancer treatment. Many precision drugs are biological agents – drugs that are produced from natural sources of biological material – as opposed to traditional drugs that are chemically synthesized and are much more expensive to develop and produce. Pharma relies on the fact that doctors (if permitted) will eagerly prescribe such drugs, regardless of cost or evidence of benefit: the medical profession has become the front-of-house sales team for the industry. Doctors' professional culture obliges them to do something – anything – rather than nothing. It is now regarded as unacceptable for a doctor to tell a patient that they can't treat their disease, particularly when that disease is cancer. Oncologists, in particular, find it almost impossible to admit to such therapeutic impotence. Some brave non-conformists do indeed come clean and have the Difficult

Conversation – the admission that nothing more can be done – but for many, the siren call of the new breakthrough, the paradigm shift, the game changer, is too powerful to resist.

Robert Weinberg is one the great figures of American cancer research. He is professor at the Massachusetts Institute of Technology Center for Molecular Oncology, and has worked for decades on the genetics of cancer. In 2014, he wrote a candid, almost confessional essay for the journal *Cell*, entitled 'Coming full circle: from endless complexity to simplicity and back again'. Weinberg charted the evolution of cancer research since the 1970s. He wrote that Nixon's War on Cancer was fuelled by the mistaken conviction that cancer was caused by infectious DNA tumour retroviruses – a common phenomenon in other animals but not, as it turned out, in humans:

> Those working on DNA tumour viruses... jumped on the bandwagon, since the war cry had expanded... In retrospect, few seemed deterred by the well-established observation that most types of human cancer did not represent communicable diseases... By the mid-1970s, with rare exception, tumour virologists had come up empty-handed in their search for human retroviruses.

In the late 1970s, a new paradigm emerged, which held that cancer was a disease caused by a small number of easily identifiable genetic mutations. Weinberg was one of this new generation of molecular biologists, who dominated cancer research in the 1980s and 1990s. Their discovery of mutations (oncogenes), such as K-ras, APC and p53, did not lead, however, to the therapeutic revolution they had imagined. In the twenty-first century, cancer research entered the era of Big Data, gathered from all the 'omes' – genomes, transcriptomes, proteomes, epigenomes, kinomes, methylomes, glycomes and matrisomes. 'Omics' now finishes the science words which once ended in 'ology'. The 'omics' era has forced researchers to accept that cancer was quite a bit more complicated than they had thought:

> Then there is the nettlesome problem of multistep tumour progression: cancer is a moving target, and whatever interactions operate at one stage of tumour progression are likely to change during the next one, so that multiple solutions will need to be worked out for individual tumours. Even within an individual tumour... analyses of tumour DNAs now indicate multiple, genetically distinct subpopulations whose representation seems to vary dramatically from one stage of tumour progression to another.
>
> The data that we now generate overwhelm our abilities of interpretation, and the attempts of the new discipline of 'systems biology' to address this shortfall have to date produced few insights into cancer biology...

The coupling between observational data and biological insight is frayed if not broken.

We lack the conceptual paradigms and computational strategies for dealing with this complexity. And equally painful, we don't know how to integrate individual data sets, such as those deriving from cancer genome analyses, with other, equally important data sets, such as proteomics [the large-scale study of proteins].

Weinberg concluded: 'We can't really assimilate and interpret most of the data that we accumulate. How will all this play out? I wouldn't pretend to know.'

Cancer medicine (oncology) has become, in the words of its own leaders, a culture of medical excess. The *Lancet Oncology* commission on 'Delivering affordable cancer care in high-income countries' was written by a group of eminent cancer researchers from around the world, and was published in 2011. The commission estimated the global economic impact of cancer at nearly $900 billion. Spending on cancer care is rising rapidly for many reasons, including 'overutilization, disincentivization driven by reimbursement rules and defensive medical practice, consumer-driven over-demand, high-cost innovation, and futile disease-directed care'. The authors concluded that the current model of cancer treatment is unsustainable:

We are increasingly faced with the question of whether

the sometimes minor benefits of proven interventions are worth the cost to individuals and society. Novel, more effective, and less toxic interventions are needed, but the price of innovation contributes further to the costs of care. We are thus at a crossroads where our choices, or refusal to make choices, have clear implications for our ability to provide care in the future.

The War on Cancer is unwinnable, but looks as if it will intensify. So far, the new genetics and molecular medicine have given us treatments of marginal benefit at huge cost. As a society, we have unquestioningly accepted this cost, believing that any advance – no matter how small – in this war of attrition is worth achieving. The cost, however, is too high, and the war is unsustainable.

9

CONSUMERISM, THE NHS AND THE 'MATURE CIVILIZATION'

The NHS Cancer Drugs Fund was created by consumerist demand; this consumerism is slowly destroying Britain's most beloved institution. As I write, the NHS is marking – not really celebrating – its seventieth birthday, and the British acknowledge that it is in trouble. The onward march of the culture of medical excess, combined with a larger, older and frailer population, has led many to conclude that the service, and its foundation model, are no longer sustainable. Enoch Powell predicted this in 1966 in his book *A New Look at Medicine and Politics*. Powell is generally unknown to people under the age of fifty, proof of his own dictum that all political careers end in failure. With his precise antique diction, delivered in an incantatory Black Country-accented voice, he sounded like a relic of the Victorian Age. For most of those familiar with his name, the only thing they can recall about him is the 'rivers of blood' speech from April 1968, his denunciation of black immigration and the Race Relations Bill. An intellectual at a time when politician-intellectuals were still a feature of British public life, Powell was too idiosyncratic and too much his own man to make it to the very top. He did, however, hold ministerial office, as financial secretary to the Treasury (1957–8) and health minister (1960–3). His short book, written in the elegant style of the classicist, was on his experience as health minister. The book is regarded by many as one of the best ever written on the NHS. It is as relevant now as it was in 1966.

Although Powell's successors as health secretary have been uninspiring, I have sympathy for them because, as he so eloquently explained, demand is infinite: 'The vulgar assumption is that there is a definable amount of medical care "needed", and if that "need" was met, no more would be demanded. This is absurd. Every advance in medical science creates new needs that did not exist until the means of meeting them came into existence.' There will never be a time when the public and the health professions will agree that spending on health has reached an adequate level. The founders of the NHS naively believed that free health care would lead to a healthier populace, which would eventually lead to ever-decreasing demand for its services. Powell pointed out the error of this belief, and anticipated Ivan Illich, who later coined the phrase 'Sisyphus syndrome' to mean that the more health care given to a population, the greater their demand for care. The combination of technological change and rising expectation has driven ever-increasing spending on health care.

The word 'rationing' has traditionally been banned by British health secretaries, but Powell argued that rationing was inevitable:

> In brutal simplicity, it has to be rationed... The task is not made easier by the political convention that the existence of any rationing at all must be strenuously denied. The public are encouraged to believe that rationing in medical care was banished by the National Health Service, and that the very idea of rationing being applied to medical care is immoral and repugnant... The worst kind of rationing is that which is unacknowledged; for it is the essence of a good rationing system to be intelligible and consciously accepted.

How do we divide this limited sum equitably? Enoch Powell respected the British electorate, and did not attempt to delude or patronize them, but many of his political successors did. Beginning in the late 1980s with the Thatcher administration, successive Conservative and Labour governments have persuaded the users of the NHS that there is no rationing of health care, and that the service can be both free and run on consumerist principles of choice and service user satisfaction. From Kenneth Clarke, all health secretaries have advocated for greater patient choice. The moral philosopher Robin Downie has argued that consumerism in health care is incompatible with a publicly funded service. He pointed out that in a traditional consumer–seller interaction, the purchaser, having been given adequate information, bears the responsibility for the choice. But 'this situation does not apply in medicine. In law it is the doctor who carries the responsibility. In other words, the locus of responsibility in the two contexts of consumerism and medical professionalism are incompatible.'

There is a consensus among politicians and society at large that health spending will have to keep rising, year after year, above inflation. Powell pointed out that this was nonsensical and unsustainable. Nowadays, however, not even the most free-marketeer Tory would dare agree. This consensus is now unquestioned, although deep down the British public, and their public representatives, despite all their loud protestations of loyalty to the NHS, know that the current model cannot continue. Health care will consume an ever-greater portion of public funds, leaving less and less for housing, transport, education and (God help us) the arts. The NHS was founded, in part, because of the simple insight, after the Second World War, that if Britain could mobilize an emergency medical service during wartime, then the same organization and social co-operation could just as easily be brought to the establishment of a peacetime health service.

The consummate don and committee-man Noel Annan observed in *Our Age*: 'During the war people had observed the decencies of equal treatment… As in war, no queue-jumping. Accept your rations.' The moral foundation of the NHS was the 1942 report by William Beveridge, which identified the five 'Giant Evils' of squalor, ignorance, want, idleness and disease. Clement Attlee and Aneurin Bevan envisaged the Welfare State as a two-way social contract between government and people. Addressing the Fabian Society in 1950, Bevan warned that the National Health Service came with new responsibilities, and would demand that its users behave with responsibility, prudence and a sense of the greater good. Britain would not be a 'mature civilization', he said, 'until we have produced a citizenry which is capable not only of selections but of rejections; which says not only who goes at the head of the queue, but who goes right at the bottom of the queue.' His 'mature civilization' has not materialized, and the citizenry has ignored its moral obligation. Now, government and people collude in a mutual deception: that spending on health can and should continue to rise indefinitely, and that this service, while continuing to be free to all users, should offer the same choice and customer service as a private enterprise. This deception is now being painfully exposed.

Powell believed that a nationalized health service, free at the point of consumption, subject to infinite demand, was inherently flawed, but acknowledged that there was no political or public appetite for any alternative. He argued that these flaws were not blemishes which could be 'reformed away'. 'The Service', wrote the economist John Jewkes in a review of Powell's book in 1966, 'was based upon national self-deception, the belief that everybody can be provided with unlimited supplies of the highest quality of medical care.' The public and politicians continue to subscribe to this consumerist fallacy, although both, deep down, know it is a lie. The internal market, introduced by Margaret Thatcher, was based on two assumptions: the first – that the NHS was a monolithic bureaucracy – was true; the second – that health care would benefit from competition – was false. Far from reducing red tape, the internal market led to increases in administration costs; around 10 per cent of the NHS's annual budget is now spent on running this internal market. Labour was initially opposed to the internal market, but when Tony Blair came into power, New Labour expanded it. Many new hospitals were built as private finance initiative (PFI) schemes, the bill for which is projected to exceed the original capital cost seven-fold. The money wasted on PFI schemes would have paid the entire NHS budget for two years. The investment bankers, construction firms, commercial lawyers and management consultants have been the main beneficiaries. Hospitals were encouraged to become 'foundation trusts', which are paid by activity, rather than by annual fixed budget; administration and transaction costs are significantly higher. The 'revolving door' between government and the private sector ensured that this model has prospered – the British people have been the victims of a vast politico-commercial swindle. They are both sentimentally attached to the NHS and fed up with it. They know that something has to change, but there is no political or public appetite for this difficult conversation. Richard Smith explained the stark choices which a 'mature civilization' would have to make:

> 'The best health-care system in the world', which politicians in every country promise, will not be one that provides everything for everybody but rather one that determines what that society wants to spend on health care and then provides explicitly limited, evidence-based services in a humane and open way without asking the impossible of its staff.

What is the best model for health care? The Nobel Laureate economist Kenneth Arrow argued that the normal rules of a market do not apply to health care. In his paper 'Uncertainty and the Welfare Economics of Medical Care', published in the *American Economic Review* in 1963, Arrow wrote: 'The special economic problems of medical care can be explained as adaptations to the existence of uncertainty in the incidence of disease and the efficacy of treatment.' His fellow economist and Nobel Laureate Paul Krugman expressed it better:

> There are two distinctive aspects of health care. One is that you don't know when or whether you'll need care –

but if you do, the care can be extremely expensive. The big bucks are in triple coronary bypass surgery, not routine visits to the doctor's office; and very, very few people can afford to pay major medical costs out of pocket. This tells you right away that health care can't be sold like bread. It must be largely paid for by some kind of insurance. And this in turn means that someone other than the patient ends up making decisions about what to buy. Consumer choice is nonsense when it comes to health care. And you can't just trust insurance companies either – they're not in business for their health, or yours.

... The second thing about health care is that it's complicated, and you can't rely on experience or comparison shopping. ('I hear they've got a real deal on stents over at St Mary's!') That's why doctors are supposed to follow an ethical code, why we expect more from them than from bakers or grocery store owners... Between these two factors, health care just doesn't work as a standard market story.

Who should provide health care – the market or the state? The answer, predictably, lies somewhere in the middle. Many European countries manage demand by their use of sometimes complex systems of co-payments. The French model of health care funded by income-based social insurance is rated by the WHO as the best health-care system in the world. The post-war establishment of this system was inspired by the same Beveridge Report which laid the foundations for the NHS, but provision is both public and private. The German system has a complex mix of public and private insurance. The late German-American health economist Uwe Reinhardt argued that the German model was ideal 'because it blends a private health-care delivery system with universal coverage and social solidarity'. (Reinhardt helped devise a new health system for Taiwan; this system now covers the entire population and costs 6.6 per cent of the nation's GDP – about a third of what the US spends.) Both the French and German systems spend more than the NHS but less than the US, and both are superior, in terms of patient satisfaction and measures such as cancer survival, to the UK and the US. The French and German systems have their flaws: the French population is hugely over-medicated, while health care in Germany is highly consumerist and constitutes about a quarter of the entire economy.

I last attended the United European Gastroenterology annual meeting in 2014 in Vienna. The conference attracted 13,000 gastroenterologists and was held in a vast neo-brutalist concrete building in the city's northern suburbs. Many – like me – were there to fulfil certain professional educational requirements, in this case, the metric known as 'external' hours. The Royal College of Physicians of Ireland will only re-credential me if I spend a few days every year in neo-brutalist conference centres. Conferences like these are of real interest only to the small group of academic and medico-political players; the rest of us are registration-fee fodder, there to make up the numbers and collect our educational points. The scientific sessions are dull affairs, but these gatherings are sometimes interesting from an anthropological point of view. Medicine being an enthusiastic early adopter of new technology, I found that all questions addressed to speakers at the end of a talk or lecture had to be submitted via smartphone, which excluded me from any such dialogue. One of the main ('plenary') sessions was called: 'Healthcare in Europe 2040: Scenarios and Implications for Digestive and Liver Diseases', where three possible future scenarios were presented. I was interested to see that the project had been carried out in conjunction with a management consultancy firm called NormannPartners UK ('Strategy Consulting for a Networked World'), who market themselves as modern soothsayers and diviners of the future. I wondered what portion of my registration fee was given to this firm and what fate had placed me in the dust of clinical medicine, instead of the marble halls of NormannPartners.

NormannPartners came up with three scenarios or ages that might play out by 2040: ice, silicon and gold. During the Ice Age, Europe becomes impoverished due to depletion of natural resources, climate change and economic crisis. The European Union collapses, as does public health care. The rich are well looked after by a private health-care system, and the poor are left to fend for themselves. In the Silicon Age, there is growth of both the population (from non-EU immigration) and technology, with widespread use of social media and 'E-medicine', and with doctors working increasingly as advisors. In the Golden Age, there is a United Europe, with universal access to health care, and a single homogenized health-care system across the continent. The snazzy booklet has a timeline chart for each possible scenario. I have looked again very carefully, but it seems NormannPartners UK (who are London-based) did not anticipate Brexit, which rather questions their credentials as predictors of the future. Ireland, where I live and work, already has an Ice Age Health Service; I won't have to wait until 2040. In Britain, the Brexiteer politicians promised their electorate that withdrawal from the EU would free up an extra £350 million every week for the NHS. They now concede that this was untrue. More importantly, Britain has lost its best chance of health reform by leaving the EU. There will be no Golden Age – except for strategy consultants.

Aneurin Bevan established the NHS without the assistance of strategy consultants – although Lord Moran (president of the Royal College of Physicians and Churchill's private physician) smoothed the way for him with the medical profession. Bevan was born in Tredegar in South Wales; he started work as a miner at the local colliery at the age of thirteen. The Medical Aid Society set up by the miners' unions in South Wales inspired Bevan to extend free health care to the entire nation. Launching the NHS, Bevan said: 'All I am doing is extending to the entire population of Britain the benefits we had in Tredegar for a generation or more. We are going to "Tredegarise" you.' The novelist A. J. Cronin worked as a GP in Tredegar in the 1920s ('Aberlaw' in *The Citadel*); he was less enamoured than Bevan of the Miners' Medical Aid Society: 'There is certainly value in the scheme... but it also has its own defects, of which the chief one, in Tredegar, was this – with complete *carte blanche* in the way of medical attention, the people were not sparing by day or night, in "fetching the doctor".'

The consumerist ethos is at the heart of the new model of the doctor–patient relationship. According to Dr Catherine Calderwood, the chief medical officer for Scotland, 'the future model of care is one with an empowered patient in a shared decision-making partnership with the clinician'. She argues that the paternalistic era of 'Doctor knows best' is over, and that the doctor–patient relationship must change. Her suggestions include 'more engaging multimedia formats', audio recordings of consultations, and the use of 'navigators', advocates who explore with patients what is important to them in terms of quality of life, life expectancy and side effects. 'Catering for this new type of relationship with our empowered "Google generation"', she says, 'is one of our biggest challenges.' Dr Calderwood's professional background is in obstetrics, where most of her patients are in their twenties and thirties. One of her civil servants might have gently pointed out to her that those most in need of health care – the elderly – do not regard themselves as part of the

'Google generation', and are not particularly interested in 'engaging, multimedia formats'.

Contemporary commentators such as Catherine Calderwood use the word 'paternalism' in an exclusively pejorative way. But some older doctors, such as Bernard Lown (b. 1921), author of *The Lost Art of Healing* (1996), believe that a certain kind of paternalism gives hope and reassurance to sick people. Lown watched his mentor Samuel Levine conclude every consultation by placing his hand on the patient's shoulder, telling them – regardless of their problem or prognosis – 'you'll be fine'. The gesture and words were so powerful that Lown used them throughout his forty-five-year career.

Consumerism has created patients who confuse needs and wants, and who often want the wrong things; it has created doctors who view medicine not as a profession, but as a service industry. Aneurin Bevan challenged the British people to take on the moral responsibilities that came with the NHS. These responsibilities included utility – the maximizing of benefit for the majority of the population – and equity: 'My Methodist parents used to say, "Have the courage my son, to say 'No'." Well, it takes a good deal of courage, but we shall have to say "No" more and more, because only by saying "No" more and more to many things can you say "Yes" to the most valuable things.' But neither politicians nor people were equal to this challenge; the Thatcherite consensus prevailed over Bevan's grand vision of a 'mature civilization'.

10

QUANTIFIED, DIGITIZED
AND FOR SALE

The American rich can now access a new type of hyper-consumerist health care, a model they present to the rest of the world as how medicine really should be. The biotechnology entrepreneur Craig Venter is in the vanguard of this movement. He is most famous for the bitterly contested race his company, Celera, fought against the publicly funded consortium headed by Francis Collins to be the first to map the human genome. Venter was later sacked by Celera, and now heads a venture called Human Longevity, Inc.™ (HLI). He has set up a clinic, the Health Nucleus, where, for $25,000, you can have your genome and microbiome (the bugs in your gut) characterized, along with a total body MRI, bone-density scanning, hundreds of blood tests, analysis of cognitive function, and so on. Google's director of engineering, Ray Kurzweil, who believes in a future where humans will become immortal, is one of HLI's advisors. Although Venter is planning to expand HLI's customer base, for the moment the market is the wealthy, for whom the promise of health is 'the ultimate luxury item'. HLI is slowly building a database from these rich consumers, linking their fully sequenced genomes with all the other phenotypic and clinical data gathered by the $25,000 'physical'. Venter, whose long-term plan is to sell these data to pharmaceutical and insurance companies and health-care providers, is admired as a pioneer of 'digital health'.

Digital health, also known by a slew of catchy phrases such as 'E-medicine', 'eHealth', 'Medicine 2.0', 'iMedicine' and 'Health 2.0', is an umbrella term used to describe a number of new technology-driven developments in medicine. These include the use of biosensors to monitor health, tele-medicine – carrying out medical consultations via digital media, the digitization of individuals' genomes, and the use of social media to create 'communities' of patients. Digital health appeals mainly to those who need health care the least: the young and the rich. It is driven by a new cadre of techno-utopians, who proclaim themselves as 'creative disrupters' of the old order. Enthusiasts argue that digital health will empower the patient, end the traditional patriarchalism of the medical profession and drive down the costs of health care. There is political support for digital health: the US Affordable Care Act ('Obamacare') promotes tele-consultations and patient self-monitoring. The surgeon and former junior health minister Lord Ara Darzi, in his 2018 report on NHS funding, warns that 'having grown up in the age of the Internet, artificial intelligence and Big Data they [the next generation] will not stand for an analogue health and care service.' Darzi is particularly entranced by the 'convergence revolution', a phrase which emerged from the Massachusetts Institute of Technology (MIT) in 2011, and which modestly announced itself as 'the third revolution in life sciences'. A 2016 report from MIT claims that 'truly major advances in the fight against cancer, dementia and diseases of aging, still rampant infectious disease, and a host of other pressing health challenges will only come from a novel research strategy that integrates biomedical knowledge with advanced engineering skills and expertise from physical, computational and mathematical sciences, an approach known as Convergence.'

Digital health has been described as a paradigmatic shift from 'mechanical' medicine to 'informational' medicine, with the focus on generating data from the human body. Techno-boosters routinely use the phrase 'digitizing the body'. The American cardiologist Eric Topol is one of the leading 'creative disrupters'. A classic Cartesian, Topol proposes a new bio-digital model, which he calls the Human GIS (Geographic Information System), consisting of multiple 'omes': phenome, genome, transcriptome, microbiome, epigenome, and so on. Technology already available on smartphones allows us to monitor all sorts of physiological variables, such as heart

rhythm and blood glucose, and Topol boasts that he pre-
scribes more apps than drugs. His brand of digital health is
unashamedly consumerist: Topol's bestselling book on the
subject is entitled *The Patient Will See You Now* – implying
an upending of the old power imbalance between patient
and doctor.

Digital health is big business: the global market for wearable self-tracking technologies was worth $3.2 billion in 2014,
with an expectation to grow to $18.8 billion in 2019. Ameri-
can corporations see these tracking devices as a means of
reducing their spending on health insurance for their employees. The retail company Target offered 335,000 Fitbit fitness-
tracker devices to its US workers; the oil company BP had a
similar offer. The Affordable Care Act allows companies to
reduce the cost of health insurance premiums by up to 30 per
cent when workers participate in such 'corporate wellness
plans'. Eric Topol doesn't see any downside to corporations
monitoring their employees: 'There are data suggesting that
when good behaviour, such as exercise, is fun and "gami-
fied", it's particularly well received and motivating... British Petroleum and Autodesk are large companies that have
incorporated wearable sensors for their employee base,
initially tracking exercise and sleep.' It is highly likely that
in the near future – particularly in the US – employees of
major corporations will be required to wear digital devices
which track their health and their behaviour. This is already
happening on a voluntary basis, with a variety of incentives,

but will soon become compulsory. Those who refuse to co-operate with this surveillance will become the new uninsured health underclass.

Another strand of digital health is online patient communities such as PatientsLikeMe. This online community was launched in 2006 by Jamie and Ben Heywood after their brother Stephen was diagnosed with motor neurone disease. Eric Topol is a great supporter: 'The pervasive progression towards openness is fuelling a remarkable degree of activism across consumers, patient groups, research foundations, and the life science industry.' When I looked up the website of PatientsLikeMe, I found that this 'community' seemed very much like any other for-profit tech company, with pictures of smiling vice presidents for 'Innovation' and 'Computational Biology'. The website states: 'Our goal is to make as much data as possible openly accessible to researchers, and to you.' PatientsLikeMe encourages members to 'donate' their health data, and to resist 'the culture of distrust towards pharmaceutical companies'. The company freely admits that it sells health data gathered from its members to pharmaceutical companies. In 2010, PatientsLikeMe was the target of data 'scraping' by the informatics and media company Nielsen; PatientsLikeMe chairman Jamie Heywood told the *Wall Street Journal*: 'We're a business, and the reality is that someone came in and stole from us.' A digital pharma stealth economy has emerged with companies like PatientsLikeMe who monetize the sick while promising to 'empower' them. There are now numerous 'disease awareness communities', many on Facebook and YouTube; members of these 'unbranded' communities may not be aware that the 'moderators' are paid by pharmaceutical corporations.

Genomics is the great hope of digital health. For more than a decade now, companies such as 23andMe have offered direct-to-consumer genetic testing, the cost of which has fallen steadily. The service was initially gimmicky, telling customers why they had dry earwax or smelled asparagus in their urine, but over the years became more serious, advising users on their risk of diabetes, dementia and various cancers. 23andMe engaged in a long dispute with the US Food and Drug Administration (FDA). The FDA clearly had serious concerns about 23andMe's methods, and in 2013 ordered the company to stop marketing its saliva-collection kits and Personal Genome Service. After prolonged negotiations, the FDA finally granted approval. Many of 23andMe's customers are so frightened by their test results (for example, a 60 per cent risk of developing Alzheimer's disease with two copies of the ApoE4 variant gene) that genetic counsellors cannot keep pace with the demand for their services.

Anne Wojcicki, CEO of 23andMe, has stated that her ambition is to build a database with the DNA data from 25 million customers: 'An incredibly valuable tool for all research – for academics, for pharma companies.' The science writer Charles Seife has written that 23andMe's long-term ambition is the same as Google and Facebook:

The Personal Genome Service isn't primarily intended to be a medical device. It is a mechanism meant to be a front end for a massive information-gathering operation against an unwitting public... For 23andMe's Personal Genome Service is much more than a medical device; it is a one-way portal into a world where corporations have access to the innermost contents of your cells and where insurers and pharmaceutical firms and market-ers might know more about your body than you know yourself. And as 23andMe warns on its website, 'genetic information that you share with others could be used against your interests. You should be careful about shar-ing your Genetic Information with others.'

Facebook and Google also started out with similar rhetoric about 'empowering' consumers and creating 'communities'. Anne Wojcicki was once married to Google's Sergey Brin. At a TED meeting in 2014, Brin's business partner and Google co-founder Larry Page said: 'Wouldn't it be amazing to have anonymous medical records available to all research doctors? Making our medical records open for sharing would save 100,000 lives a year.' (Quite how Page arrived at this figure is not clear.) Eric Topol approvingly quotes a medical software expert, Melissa McCormack, who suggests that 'we'd all be better off with our health records on Facebook'. It is not difficult to predict where the digital health movement is heading. Companies such as 23andMe will harvest huge numbers of individual genomes. This information will be purchased, directly or indirectly, by pharma, health insurance companies and other agencies, including life insurance companies, potential employers and government agencies. Harvard University's Personal Genome Project (PGP) requires volunteers to consent to sharing of their data: 'The PGP', writes Eric Topol, 'has leveraged online forums, LinkedIn and Facebook, along with annual meetings, to provide a highly interactive experience and education for the participants who are largely without a background in science.' The Global Alliance for Genomics and Health (GA4GH) held its first meeting in 2014, where 150 organizations were represented, including Google.

The Orwellian dystopia is well under way: a US start-up called Miinome pays poor people cash for their genome. An American company called Exact Data sells lists of people with sexually transmitted diseases. The Carolinas Health System mines consumer credit card data to identify high-risk patients, through their purchases of alcohol, tobacco and other unhealthy items. In 2013, the UK government launched a major campaign called Care.data: the medical history of all NHS patients was digitized and stored in a central repository at the Health and Social Care Information Centre (HSCIC). In February 2014, data on 47 million patients was sold to an insurance company. The trade in medical data is big business. Data brokers such as the US firm IMS Health collect data from pharmacies and insurance companies; it sells information to pharma on the prescribing habits of individual doctors to help these companies refine their marketing. Pfizer spends $12 million every year on health data from companies like IMS. Other buyers include advertising companies and institutional investors in pharma. Medical data are never 'private': data-mining tools used by companies like IMS can easily crack supposedly anonymous databases by cross-referencing data from other sources. IMS say they have no commercial incentive to identify specific individuals, but other data brokers will surely figure out how individuals' data can be monetized. The digital health techno-utopians view privacy as quaint, old-fashioned and redundant, an obstacle to 'sharing' data with industrial 'partners'. Some have gone further, arguing that privacy as a notion is now opposed to the collective good and is therefore not only out-dated, but positively antisocial. Facebook and Google make money by monetizing their users, by extracting and selling their data. At present, these tech giants mine the Little Data, but what they are really interested in is the Big Data, and what could be bigger than the genome, and all the other 'omes' that make up a human being?

Online medical consultation services are now well estab-lished, and appeal mainly to the young. Many have expressed concern about the absence of regulation, lack of continuity and inappropriate prescribing; traditional doctors baulk at the idea of treating patients without carrying out a physical examination. But the physical examination has lost its importance; doctors now spend more time staring at screens than they do looking at patients. US medical students and trainees have become so detached from the basics of medicine that the physician and novelist Abraham Verghese (who works at Stanford Medical School) has rebranded the physical examination as the 'Stanford 25': 'twenty-five technique-dependent, physical diagnosis manoeuvres'. Although I am suspicious of the phrase 'Stanford 25' – implying, as it does, that Stanford Medical School somehow invented the physical examination – Verghese has correctly argued that the ritual and physical contact of the physical examination are a vital component of that unquantifiable thing called 'healing'. Many within American medicine lament the obsession with digital data at the expense of old-fashioned doctoring. John Mandrola, a cardiologist, wrote:

> As the healthcare machine increasingly embraces mobile sensors, digital records, and binary quality metrics, what used to be the care of people has tragically become the treatment of aberrations of 1s and 0s.
>
> … Good doctoring is not rocket science. But it is also not digital. It is not a white screen. It is not numbers from a pulmonary artery. And it does not come quickly. It requires seeing patients alongside mentors over years. What worries me is that we are taking our eyes and ears off people. We are distracted, perhaps intoxicated, by the 1s and 0s.

Eric Topol views doctors like me as the chief professional obstacle to digital health: 'Half of American physicians are over age fifty-five, far removed from digital native status (under age 30).' Topol (sixty-four), with his 2.8 million Instagram followers, is the disco-dancing dad of digital health. The self-styled 'medical futurist', the Hungarian Bertalan Meskó, is Topol's ideal digital native doctor: 'Since the age of fourteen, I have been logging details of my life every single day. It means not one day is missing from my digital diary which now consists of over 6,600 days with data.' Like Topol, he argues that 'the ivory tower of medicine is no more', and that 'patients, now called e-patients or empowered patients, who are ready to hack and disrupt healthcare need guidance.'

There have been several recent examples of digital snake oil, the most conspicuous being Theranos, a health technology firm founded in 2003 by a nineteen-year-old Stanford dropout called Elizabeth Holmes. Her idea was to sell cheap blood tests by the attractive gimmick of taking a tiny drop of blood, run it through the nanotechnology called 'lab on a chip' and return hundreds of results in minutes. She described this as 'the iPod of health care'. Holmes, good-looking and charismatic, was a brilliant saleswoman and persuaded very rich people such as Rupert Murdoch to invest in Theranos, which at its peak was valued at $10 billion. Two former US secretaries of state – George Shultz and Henry Kissinger – were persuaded to join the board of directors. Holmes negotiated a contract with the pharmacy giant Walgreen, and all 8,200 drugstores in the chain had a 'Theranos corner'. John Carreyrou, a Pulitzer Prize-winning investigative journalist with the *Wall Street Journal*, was alerted by a whistle-blower that all was not what it seemed at Theranos. He found that the technology wasn't accurate and had never undergone independent testing. Holmes and Theranos responded with a campaign of legal intimidation described as 'vicious', but Carreyrou and the *Wall Street Journal* stood up to this charismatic bully. Theranos's share price collapsed, and they were sued by Walgreen. In June 2018, Holmes and her business partner Sunny Balwani were indicted on multiple counts of fraud. Eric Topol was entranced by Holmes: 'She gets it – she's a digital native'; he lauded her rhetoric about a patient's access to their blood tests being 'a basic human right'. When Holmes was found out, Topol wrote a self-serving new epilogue to his book *The Patient Will See You Now*, in which he stated: 'I remained concerned about the total lack of transparency of the company's technology.'

Digital health originated in part from the Quantified Self movement, whose motto is 'self-knowledge through numbers'. This movement was founded in 2007 by Kevin Kelly and Gary Wolf of *Wired* magazine. The Quantified Self – and digital health – are symptoms of the contemporary obsession with control. Data and metrics are regarded as clean and predictable, far removed from the contingencies of real life and the messiness and uncertainty of the body and its ailments. Although it was first coined by the American author David Brooks, the Israeli historian Yuval Noah Harari has popularized the word 'Dataism' to describe this modern pseudo-religion:

> Like every religion, it has its practical commandments. First and foremost, a Dataist ought to maximise data flow by connecting to more and more media, and producing and consuming more and more information. Like other successful religions, Dataism is also missionary. Its second commandment is to connect everything to the system, including heretics who don't want to be connected.

Digital health also reflects a global societal shift towards neoliberal values of self-responsibility for health maintenance, along with a decline in state-provided health and social care. Americans have enthusiastically embraced digital health because they believe it will reduce their ever-rising, and out of control, spending on health. The overwhelming likelihood is that it will do the exact opposite: historically, new technology has always driven up the cost of health care. So far, the chief beneficiaries have been the medical–industrial complex and the technology corporations.

Digital health is the logical conclusion of Ivan Illich's 'social iatrogenesis' – the wider cultural harm (as distinct to harm inflicted on individuals) caused by medicine's hegemony – and Petr Skrabanek's 'coercive healthism'. Both would have been grimly satisfied that they have been proved right: digital health will create a surveillance society, or 'data dictatorships', as Yuval Noah Harari predicts. In his book *The Death of Humane Medicine*, published shortly before his death in 1994, Skrabanek warned:

> In the iatrocratic state (to use Thomas Szasz's term), power is vested in the priests of the body and the priests of the mind. 'Health' is the supreme virtue and must be maintained at all costs. Every person, without realizing it, writes his or her own dossier, where every deviation from the norm is recorded at regular screenings. Notes are taken on lifestyle, risk factors and genetic profile. The doctor, the employer, the insurance company and the police hold (or soon will hold) in their interlinked computers all the information required, according to which the person will be judged when applying for a job, seeking medical care, applying for medical insurance, intending to travel abroad or wishing to procreate. With healthism as a state ideology, the blueprint for the iatrocratic state exists. It is being implemented by degrees. This book is intended as a warning.

Neither Illich nor Skrabanek anticipated, however, that coercion would not be needed: the new 'e-patients' have willingly and happily handed themselves over. Skrabanek died before the Internet really got going, and well before the arrival of the tech giants. Healthism now is not predominantly coercive, imposed by the state with an agenda of social engineering, but a broad societal consensus that more medicine, more health care, is good. The tech corporations and the medical–industrial complex will round up vast populations who will not resist, who are happy to be herded because they are assured that they are empowered members of a digital, and digitized, community.

11

THE ANTI-HARLOTS

Consumerist movements like digital health have the explicit aim of reducing the power of doctors and rebalancing the doctor–patient relationship in the patient's favour. The power of doctors, however, has been in steady decline for decades. After the Bristol and Shipman scandals, British doctors were subjected to a degree of scrutiny and regulation endured by no other professional group. This new regulation was initially ordered by politicians such as Alan Milburn and judges such as Dame Janet Smith; the General Medical Council and the Royal Colleges all eagerly co-operated. I left the NHS just in time – in 2001 – but Ireland is following close behind, as it always does.

When I qualified in 1983, I caught the end of the golden era of the medical profession and of medical innovation. The decades since then have witnessed numerous NHS scandals.

In the ten years from 1998 to 2008 alone there were four: Bristol, Alder Hey, Shipman and Stafford. The Bristol Royal Infirmary Inquiry was set up in 1998 under the chairmanship of Ian Kennedy QC to investigate the deaths of children who had undergone cardiac surgery there. The inquiry's report was published in 2001 and was severely critical of the surgeons' performance and professional culture. The Kennedy report recommended the introduction of regular appraisal and revalidation for doctors. One of the senior surgeons, James Wisheart, and the chief executive, Dr John Roylance, were struck off by the General Medical Council. One of the witnesses to the Bristol inquiry drew attention to the large number of children's hearts stored in the pathology department at Alder Hey Hospital in Liverpool. This led to another report, published in 2001, which caused a national outcry and eventually led to the Human Tissue Act in 2004. In 2000, the Manchester-based GP Harold Shipman was found guilty of murdering fifteen patients. An inquiry was set up in 2001 under the chairmanship of Dame Janet Smith, and reported in 2005. The report recommended much tighter regulation of doctors. The greatest NHS scandal, however, concerned the care of patients and mortality rates at Stafford Hospital. The story broke in 2007 and led to two public inquiries chaired by Robert Francis QC, a barrister specializing in medical law.

The power and prestige of the medical profession ebbed away. This loss was both self-inflicted and the result of various unforeseen events and societal changes. These events include the scandals listed above, the Internet, and the increasing politicization and monetization of health care. The medical profession sleepwalked through all of this, ceding leadership to managers and Big Science academics. Drastic and catastrophic changes to working practices, and the protocolization of care were accepted with barely a whimper. In the NHS, the scandals from Bristol onwards made it easy for the politicians and the managers, ably assisted by the judiciary and the media, to strip away this power. I do not mean to glamorize the world of my youth. It would be disingenuous of me to argue that doctors were better in 1983. They weren't. I worked for men (they were mainly men) who were greedy, lazy, arrogant and incompetent. I also worked for men who were selfless, devoted to their patients and kind to their juniors and students. I am unconcerned by status for its own sake, but status should at least be commensurate with responsibility. We handed over our power but not our accountability to our patients. Stanley Baldwin famously dismissed the press as exercising 'power without responsibility – the prerogative of the harlot throughout the ages'. Doctors have become anti-harlots: we carry responsibility without exercising power.

The philosopher Ronald Dworkin wrote of the professional autonomy once enjoyed by doctors: 'They did not have to be backslappers or joke-tellers or handshakers; they did not have to get along with their boss or be shrewdly political. Their healing skill was enough to attract patients and earn a comfortable living. Their job in life was largely to supervise themselves. They answered to no one but their patients.' But that changed too: we're all in sales now. Perhaps doctors no longer command respect because they have ceased to respect themselves. This manifests in little things, such as how they dress. Most hospitals now operate a 'bare below the elbows' policy, which is justified on the basis that it prevents doctors spreading hospital-acquired infections such as methicillin-resistant staphylococcus aureus (MRSA) to their patients. There is little or no evidence to support this. The NHS banned the wearing of white coats by doctors in 2008; this was essentially a political gesture, following rising public concern about hospital-acquired infection. This cheap gimmick was meant to deflect public attention from the real causes of hospital-acquired infection, such as overcrowding, shortage of single rooms and isolation facilities, the outsourcing of cleaning to the private sector, and inadequate staffing. The removal of the white coat was a political act, taking away what some saw as an outdated symbol of doctors' power. The white coat was a vestige of the golden age, associated with professional competence, scientific progress and (paradoxically) cleanliness. Patients are more likely to trust doctors who look like doctors. The white coat was a uniform, which doctors wore with pride and honour, and which made them immediately identifiable to their patients.

Medicine's degeneration and corruption has been as much aesthetic and intellectual as professional and scientific. The clinician-aristocrats may have been plutocrats at the top of a feudal medical career pyramid, but they were leaders and carried the memory of their institutions. Many had style and 'bottom' – a mysterious quality, a combination of personal substance and integrity. The profession appears to be going through a crisis of bottom; doctors still publicly proclaim their love of the job, but the statistics tell a different story with a rush to retirement. Bullied by managers and frightened of their patients, overseen and regulated by an ever-increasing number of statutory bodies, we let this happen. Over my professional lifetime, we saw the disintegration of medical teams; we saw nursing evolve into a rival, rather than a complementary, profession; we saw specialist training fracture and shorten, producing new consultants who simply weren't able; we saw administrators evolve into managers, who took over the hospitals. As doctors have lost – given away would be more accurate – their power, they must pay homage to the contemporary orthodoxy that they are simply one member of a multidisciplinary team that provides care for the patient. This orthodoxy holds that no single member of this team should be dominant, or domineering, and that all decisions are reached by happy consensus. The multidisciplinary team, however, has usually vanished when something goes wrong, leaving the doctor to assume responsibility (and punishment) for whatever awfulness has happened. In the phrase of Allyson Pollock (public health academic, and director of the Institute of Health and Society), doctors 'work in teams, but are blamed as individuals'.

In their mission to increase regulation and accountability of doctors, politicians and managers were assisted by the new breed of academic bioethicists who emerged in the 1980s and 1990s. Typical of this new breed is Sir Ian Kennedy, the academic lawyer who chaired the Bristol Inquiry. Kennedy gave the Reith Lectures in 1980, taking as his theme 'Unmasking Medicine'. His vaguely leftist critique of the medical profession, which argued for patient empowerment, ironically chimed with Margaret Thatcher's plan to reform the medical profession and the NHS along consumerist lines. Education, local government and social services would be subjected to similar reforms, creating what has been called the 'audit society'. Kennedy became the quintessential medical quangocrat. One of his many recommendations relating to Bristol was the establishment of a 'system of external surveillance', which led to the foundation in 2004 of the Commission for Healthcare Audit and Inspection (CHAI). The CHAI required hospital trusts to provide them with huge quantities of data. The *Lancet* accused the CHAI of creating 'an environment of prejudice, anxiety and resignation in the workplace'. The moral philosopher Onora O'Neill used her 2002 Reith Lectures 'A Question of Trust' to argue that systems aimed at increasing accountability and regulation of professionals such as doctors had the paradoxical effect of deepening the mistrust they sought to remedy. When the CHAI was closed in 2008, Kennedy lamented that regulation was seen as 'part of the problem rather than the solution'.

The case of Harold Shipman was used to justify the new draconian regulation of doctors, although most privately acknowledged that such regulation would not prevent the emergence of the occasional rogue like Shipman. This new professional elite which emerged with the audit society came to exercise a hierarchical domination of doctors who continued to carry a degree of responsibility which this elite would never have to bear.

Following the collapse of power of the clinician-aristocrats, the vacuum was filled by managers and a new breed called clinical directors, who viewed their role through a managerialist prism. The clinical directors were distrusted by their fellow doctors and manipulated by their managers, so they never achieved the prestige of the clinician-aristocrats. Power within medicine seeped out of the hospitals to the committee rooms and the universities. The new breed of professor was a Big Science Brahmin, and the committee men and women sought prestige in the royal colleges, professional bodies and medical schools. Clinical work was strictly for the unambitious. All of this has left the hospitals essentially leaderless. Managers and clinical directors are nominally in charge, but they are motivated mainly by targets and metrics, and are unconcerned with maintaining the 'invisible glue' which once held hospitals together. This lack of leadership, both among nurses and doctors, contributed significantly to the chaos and squalor that eventually led to the scandal at Stafford. Doctors are so divided by factional fighting and boosterism for 'our' diseases and services that we no longer function as a cohesive profession pursuing a common good. We have poisoned the well of our craft and our tradition.

The lazy stereotype of hospital consultants as pinstriped bullies has proved remarkably enduring, and impervious to the grim realities faced by contemporary doctors. Doctors now – just like their patients – are pawns in a global business. Peter Bazalgette, author of *The Empathy Instinct*, and most famous for the dubious distinction of bringing the vulgar and exploitative *Big Brother* to British television, believes doctors work in an environment as cocooned from reality as the 'housemates' on his TV show. He laments the 'tendency in doctors towards grandiosity and omnipotence', taking as his example of this tendency the fictional surgeon Sir Lancelot Spratt, played by the great James Robertson Justice in the *Doctor in the House* films, seven of which were made between 1954 and 1970. Spratt, writes Bazalgette, was 'the bombastic, aggressive, megalomaniacal surgeon... [who] harassed the nurses, terrified the junior doctors and treated the patients like unfortunate serfs'. For most of history, however, doctors were not held in high esteem, and the prestige of the profession during the golden age is probably a brief historical anomaly. From Molière to Shaw, doctors were portrayed as pompous, ignorant, greedy and useless. Ivan Illich observed that for all of history before the French Revolution, doctors earned their living as artisans. He had a low opinion of the medical profession, whom he regarded as more concerned with their income and status than the health of their patients: 'Doctors deploy themselves as they like, more so than other professionals, and they tend to gather where the climate is healthy, where the water is clean, and where people are employed and can pay for their services.' The Flexner Report (1910) into medical education in the US and Canada documented the shockingly low quality of medical education at the time. A. J. Cronin's 1937 bestseller *The Citadel* was a portrait of the lamentable standards of British medicine between the wars. The erosion of status over the last thirty years has simply put doctors back in their rightful historical place, and they are unhappy. Complaints against doctors to the General Medical Council doubled between 2007 and 2012. The NHS paid out £1.4 billion to settle medical negligence claims in 2015–16, a figure which has more than doubled in ten years. There have been several high-profile cases of doctors convicted of gross negligence manslaughter. The London surgeon David Sellu spent fifteen months in prison before having his conviction overturned on appeal. Hadiza Bawa-Garba, a paediatrician nearing the end of her training, was convicted of gross negligence man-slaughter in 2016, following the death of a six-year-old boy called Jack Adcock. Her professional training log, which encourages trainees to write 'reflections', was used in evi-dence against her. The medical profession in Britain has been outraged by the treatment of Sellu and Bawa-Garba: the mouse may yet roar.

You might argue that the happiness and morale of doctors is of no concern to anyone outside the profession and their families: this has been the view of politicians, managers and the media. A functioning health-care system, however, cannot exist without a strong and well-supported medical profession. Doctors – particularly GPs – are retiring early; a GP friend of mine quit his NHS practice in his mid-forties simply because he could no longer bear the behaviour of many of his patients. The end of deference very quickly became the start of insolence. Doctors often blame politicians, managers, journalists and lawyers for their woes. While it is true that these groups have not been well disposed to us, we have mainly ourselves to blame. We conceive of ourselves as powerless victims of uncontrollable external forces, but this is false. Our complacency and collective cowardice have placed us where we are now.

Decisions that used to be routinely taken by doctors are now often referred to the courts. The cases of Charlie Gard, Isaiah Haastrup and Alfie Evans, which have received extensive media coverage in Britain, are broadly similar. All three baby boys had severe, irreversible brain injury, and could not survive outside an intensive care unit. The doctors involved quite reasonably advised the respective parents that further intensive care was futile, and that the children should be allowed to die 'with dignity', as the trite modern formula puts it. In all three cases, the parents would not agree and exhausted every legal avenue in a battle against the doctors and hospitals. They also conducted parallel publicity campaigns via the newspapers and social media. The courts ruled in favour of the hospitals in all three cases; all three boys have since died. These cases were presented by the media as an ethical dilemma, but there was no dilemma in any case. A dilemma implies a difficult choice, picking the best, or least worst, of two or more alternatives. There was no alternative scenario in which Charlie Gard could have survived and enjoyed life outside the intensive care unit of Great Ormond Street Hospital. The problem was not an ethical one, but one of authority and expertise. Hospitals have always dealt with severely brain-damaged children and their parents. Each case, until now, was a private tragedy. The doctors and nurses did the best they could and, when the moment arrived, told the parents that it was time to let go. What has changed is the refusal of contemporary young parents to take the doctors at their word, to accept their authority and their experience. Why is this happening now? There are several reasons: the gradual disappearance of deference to professionals and authority figures; the democratization of knowledge via the Internet; the new distrust of 'experts' and the inflammatory effects of social media.

Doctors have been wrong-footed by all of this. The ortho-doxy that 'communication skills' solve all such problems has been shown to be a hollow fantasy. Many of the doctors and nurses who treated Charlie Gard received death threats and were spat at by 'supporters' of the family; some have not returned to work. Michael McDowell, the Irish barrister and former minister for justice, criticized doctors and hospitals for routinely referring cases to the High Court which they should deal with themselves. By choosing the legal route so often, doctors have tacitly conceded that they no longer have the authority – the bottom – to make, and stand by, these difficult decisions. What are they afraid of? These conflicts are now so common that professional mediators have emerged. Dr Chris Danbury, an intensive care specialist in Reading, is a registered mediator and is regularly engaged by hospitals to negotiate with families. He gives us a flavour of the challenges involved:

This [case] involved a young father in his early twenties who had an untreatable, progressive, ultimately fatal neuro-degenerative condition. He had been transferred back from his local neurosciences centre to his local hospital. The regional centre told the local hospital that he was coming back for palliative care, but had told the family that he was being transferred back to be closer to home. When the receiving intensivist talked to the family for the first time, the family became outraged at the mention of palliative care and denied that it had ever been mentioned by the neurosciences unit. By the time I visited the hospital, there was a 29,000 signature petition calling for continued treatment. The hospital was being picketed by 250 people.

After talking to the clinicians, I asked to speak to the family. Initially hostile to the idea, they finally agreed. I then had to persuade the hospital to let me talk to the family without either police or security present. Eventually I ended up opposite 18 members of his family. Following a challenging start, I listened and talked to them for three hours. The following week, in the COP [Court of Appeal], the judge asked whether the situation could be resolved without him hearing the case. Despite the objections of the trust's barrister, the other two barristers felt that it was worth a try. As one of the experts in the case, I then spent around eight hours talking to the family and the clinical team. As the day went on, it became clear that the distance between the two sides was narrowing, and by the end a plan had been agreed by everyone. Treatment would continue, although some of the more invasive treatments (including CPR [cardiopulmonary resuscitation]) would not be offered. As a result, he went on to live for another couple of years.

Although I may not possess the saint-like patience of Chris Danbury, I have some experience of such conflicts, having spent most of 2012 engaged in prolonged disputes with two families. The struggle ended with the inevitable and unpreventable deaths of both patients. It was a wearying, dispiriting experience, which I survived only because I shared the burden with a sensible, courageous and supportive colleague.

The hospital did not have a formal process for dealing with such quarrels, so we were left isolated and unsupported. The continuous, well-meaning advice from the Clinical Risk Department was to organize Another Meeting: it seemed inconceivable to them that such difficulties could not be overcome by Another Meeting and what they like to call Effective Communication Skills. But, as the doctors at Great Ormond Street Hospital (Charlie Gard), King's College Hospital (Isaiah Haastrup) and Alder Hey Hospital (Alfie Evans) found out, meetings, mediation and communication skills have their limits.

The unwritten social contract between patients and doctors has broken down, and it's time we drew up a new one. Society, however, isn't clear on what it wants from doctors. Our patients want us to be simultaneously decisive yet humble, knowledgeable but not patronizing, empathetic, patient, available (both physically and psychologically), and so on. It would be difficult to find a single individual who embodies all of these qualities, which is why we feel a vague sense of inadequacy. We might channel some of the energy we currently devote to awareness campaigns to opening a dialogue with our patients. Richard Smith, then editor of the *British Medical Journal*, wrote about 'the bogus contract' in 2001. This contract is based on patients believing that modern medicine can do remarkable things; that doctors can easily diagnose what is wrong, know everything it's necessary to know, and can solve all problems, even social ones. Doctors know that these beliefs are childish, and that the contract is bogus. They know that modern medicine has limited powers, that it's often dangerous, that they can't solve social problems, that they don't know everything, that the only thing they really do know is how difficult many things are, and that the balance between doing good and harm is very fine. The bogus contract is the inevitable result of decades of medicalization of life. During my professional lifetime, medicine annexed old age, substance abuse and childhood behaviour. The late great historian of medicine Roy Porter wrote in *The Greatest Benefit to Mankind* (1997): 'Today's complex and confused attitudes towards medicine are the cumulative responses to a century of the growth of the therapeutic state and the medicalized society.' In the seventeen years since Smith wrote about this bogus contract, doctors' unhappiness has only deepened, and their status has drained away. Perhaps we should start awareness campaigns with slogans such as 'Medicine Has Limited Powers', 'Death Is Inevitable', 'Old Age Is Not a Disease'.

It is in everyone's interest to solve this. I am not optimistic, however, that this can be fixed because it would require the confluence of several events. The clinicians would have to wrest power back from the managers. They would have to negotiate a new concordat with the nursing profession. Medical litigation would have to change to a non-adversarial 'no-fault' compensation model. Regulatory bodies such as the General Medical Council would have to be radically reformed. Accountability would have to be realigned with power. The profession would need to open a dialogue with their patients, with society, with politicians, with the media about what medicine can and cannot do. How might such reforms be achieved? I am not optimistic that the coalface clinicians will suddenly rise up and cast off their shackles. The professional bodies are sclerotic, their only concern being self-preservation. Managers will not willingly hand over power; it will have to be taken from them. The incentives for the present system to continue are just so much greater than the incentives to reform. Most of all, medicine needs leadership, not limp-wristed virtue signalling. It is difficult to know where this is going to come from. Perhaps it is a problem for the next generation to solve.

I teach the next generation. At a recent tutorial with final-year medical students, it occurred to me that the ward where I was teaching was the same ward where I had worked as an intern in 1984. I told my tutorial group that, in that prelapsarian Eden, all my patients were on one ward – not scattered all over the hospital, or on trolleys in the emergency department. When my boss – the professor of medicine – did a ward round, he was accompanied throughout by the senior ward sister, and the round concluded in her office over tea. Perhaps the many intervening years have given an excessively rosy glow to my memories, but when I compared it to the kind of round I do now, it seems like a very heaven. Following my last weekend on-call for General Medicine, I had over fifty patients under my care, scattered across fifteen locations within the hospital. I start at 7 a.m. so the junior doctors on-call the night before can go home at 9 a.m. All of these rounds start in the emergency department, where I have ten patients: four in cubicles and six on trolleys in the corridors. Since it is so early, the corridors are dark and many of the patients are asleep. Trying to examine an elderly patient on a trolley in the corridor is quite a challenge, with the noise, the lack of privacy and the passing traffic. With each patient, the routine is the same. I get a quick summary from the junior doctor who admitted them, but very often this doctor was on an earlier shift, and has gone home. I look at the patient and decide if they are sick, or not. I write a brief note in the chart, as my conclusions are so often different from the admitting junior doctor's. I check the drug chart to see what has been prescribed. The protocols for sepsis and venous thromboembolism ensure that several patients are on intravenous antibiotics who shouldn't be, and nearly all are on an anticoagulant. I see a man in the emergency department who has had a major stomach haemorrhage. He needs an urgent endoscopy, but this cannot happen until he is allocated a bed. A twenty-two-year-old with liver cirrhosis (due to alcohol) has been admitted with jaundice and fluid retention. He will be dead within a year. A man with advanced dementia in long-term psychiatric care has been sent in with a chest infection. Because he coughs and splutters when swallowing (this is long-standing) the nurses have him assessed by a speech and language therapist who concludes

205

that the man has an 'unsafe' swallow, and cannot be allowed to eat or drink. I reverse this order, to the great relief of the patient and the annoyance of the therapist. It takes several hours to see the patients, partly because they are so scattered – this is called a 'safari' ward round. On most wards, the nurses do not accompany us, so much vital information is lost or never relayed. Over the weekend, I am obliged to join morning conference calls with the clinical director and nurse managers. Much of the discussion involves potential breaches of targets for patients accommodated on trolleys in the emergency department.

I eventually finish at 12.30 p.m., five-and-a-half hours after starting in the emergency department. Most of my patients are elderly people, many from nursing homes. Most are on several long-term medications – some are taking as many as twenty – all, no doubt, prescribed by their well-meaning GPs, who are simply following guidelines. A few of these elderly patients are under my care at least in part because of a side effect of one of these drugs. The day is one of intense pressure and concentration; clinical judgement is the principal value I bring to this round. My role is to identify the patients who have not been sorted out, whose admitting diagnosis is incorrect, who are not getting the right treatment. This judgement, in the world of protocolized, evidence-based medicine, is not highly regarded. And despite all the squalor, chaos, distraction and poor communication, the responsibility for all these patients is mine, and mine alone.

The work of the junior doctors and nurses is ruled by protocols. The nurses have 'early warning scores' which trigger
an urgent call to a doctor; most are false alarms. The junior
doctors, meanwhile, are forced by protocols to prescribe
antibiotics and anticoagulants to large numbers of patients
who do not require them, and who may suffer harm. All of
this induces a feeling of weariness and futility. The research
laboratory seems a long way from this ward round, and
evidence-based medicine, which led to the proliferation of
these protocols, has become a sulking bully. Our patients are
no longer people, but abnormal physiological and laboratory
parameters, malfunctioning organs, and what Ivan Illich
called 'bundles of diagnoses'. The doctors, nurses and other
health professionals have all done their job correctly and by
protocol. Just as the medical–industrial complex sees sick
people as malfunctioning machines, it regards doctors as
standardized and protocolized functionaries. Patients are a
problem to be processed by the hospital's conveyor belt; it
is hardly surprising that they often feel that nobody seems
to be in charge, or cares about them as individuals. My own
hospital is proud of its 'patient flow' initiative, which gives
explicit institutional approval and branding to the factory
model of health care, where sick people are a quantifiable
input that must be processed into an output, with the turn-
over ever shorter. We are treating, but we are not healing.

After the round, I retreat to my office for a sandwich, and
catch up on my emails. There is an invitation to a workshop

on 'open disclosure', an initiative aimed to diminish the fall-out from medical error by a policy of admission of culpability from the beginning. I note that none of the four 'facilitators' of this workshop is a doctor; none has had to tell a patient and a family that they have made a mistake. Another email informs me that my attendance at a training session on hand-washing is compulsory. Yet another, from my professional indemnity organization, invites me to attend workshops on mastering difficult interactions with patients and shared decision-making. A message from one of the royal colleges invites me to attend a seminar on 'leadership for clinicians'. I ponder the paradox of those shrewd doctors who escape the stresses of the clinical front line by teaching other doctors how to be leaders.

12

THE MCNAMARA FALLACY

The main ideological difference between doctors and managers is that managers believe that health care can be run like a business, and that data are the key to success: they are 'Dataists'. In a system such as the NHS, which is entirely state-funded, politicians have a duty to ensure that the service is accountable and answerable to that mythical figure, 'the tax-payer'. This not unreasonable obligation led, over many decades, to an obsession with metrics – that which is measurable. This feverish monomania created the cancerous target culture that now pervades the NHS.

Over-emphasis on metrics is often referred to as the McNamara fallacy. Robert Strange McNamara (1916–2009) was US Secretary of State from 1961 to 1968, during the presidencies of John F. Kennedy and Lyndon B. Johnson. His career was, by any standard, stellar: after graduating in economics at Berkeley, he took an MBA at the Harvard Business School, and became its youngest professor at the age of twenty-four. During the Second World War, McNamara served in the US military's Department of Statistical Control. He applied the rigorous statistical methodology which he had learned at Harvard to the planning and execution of aerial bombing missions, achieving a dramatic improvement in efficiency. McNamara served in Europe and the Far East, where he assisted General Curtis LeMay in the planning of the fire-bombing of Japanese cities, when over 100,000 civilians perished in one night. After the war, the Ford Motor Corporation recruited several members of Statistical Control, including McNamara; these clever young men were nick-named the 'whiz kids'. The once-great company was then in disarray and losing money. McNamara and his fellow whiz kids applied their skills of rational statistical analysis to the problems of the ailing giant, achieving huge improvements, and returned Ford to profit. In 1960, at the age of forty-four, he was appointed president of the Ford Corporation, the first person outside the Ford family to achieve this distinction. After less than two months in this post, McNamara was offered a cabinet position by President-elect John F. Kennedy. He rejected the initial offer of treasury secretary, believing he was not qualified for this position, but accepted the post of defense secretary.

McNamara used the same rigorous systemic analysis at the Pentagon that had worked so well at Ford, reducing costs and increasing efficiency. As the conflict in Vietnam escalated in the early 1960s, McNamara applied this quantitative approach to the prosecution of the war. He believed that as long as enemy casualties exceeded the numbers of US dead, the war would eventually be won: 'Things you can count, you ought to count; loss of life is one.' He set a figure of 250,000 enemy casualties as the 'crossover point', beyond which the North Vietnamese would be unable to replace their dead with new troops. By 1967, however, the US was no nearer to concluding the war, despite a massive increase in ground troops and aerial bombardment of North Vietnam. Public opposition to the war had grown: even McNamara's son Craig, a student at Stanford, took part in an anti-war demonstration. McNamara concluded that the conflict was unwinnable, and wrote a memo to President Johnson and the joint chiefs of staff advising de-escalation and commencement of a peace settlement. Johnson didn't reply to this memo, and in late 1967, eased McNamara out of the administration. 'I wasn't sure if I resigned or was sacked', McNamara later wrote. In April 1968 he became president of the World Bank, a position he held until 1981. Clark Clifford, who succeeded McNamara as defense secretary, observed:

Vietnam was not a management problem, it was a war, and war is about life and death, filled with intangibles that defy analysis. He [McNamara] had never been in a war, and perhaps he did not fully appreciate at first its stupid waste and its irrational emotions, and the elusiveness of facts and truth when men are dying. Nor did he fully understand the political roots of the conflict until it was too late. He had tried to master the war as he had everything else in his remarkable career, using pure intellect and his towering analytical skills – but Vietnam defied such analysis.

Three years after McNamara's resignation, the sociologist and political analyst Daniel Yankelovich (1924–2017) coined the phrase 'The McNamara Fallacy' (the Anglo-Irish author Charles Handy popularized the phrase in his 1994 book *The Empty Raincoat*, and is often erroneously credited as the originator of the concept):

> The first step is to measure whatever can easily be measured. This is OK as far as it goes. The second step is to disregard that which can't be easily measured or to give it an arbitrary quantitative value. This is artificial and misleading. The third step is to presume that what can't be measured easily really isn't important. This is blindness. The fourth step is to say that what can't be easily measured really doesn't exist. This is suicide.

Medicine is, and always has been, messy, imprecise and uncertain; the McNamara fallacy is the delusion that all of this complexity can yield itself to numerical analysis. This leads to over-reliance on crude metrics, such as hospital mortality rates, and the setting of arbitrary targets, many or most of which do not improve patient care, and some of which cause harm. Meanwhile, unquantifiable attributes, such as continuity of care and compassion, are neglected.

Professor Sir Brian Jarman is British medicine's Robert McNamara. In the 1990s, he developed a new metric, the Hospital Standardized Mortality Ratio (HSMR). This metric was the single biggest factor which precipitated the scandal at Stafford Hospital, still regarded as the greatest catastrophe in the history of the NHS. Even the name 'Stafford' is now used as a kind of short-hand to encapsulate everything that is wrong with hospital care in Britain. The scandal was created by a unique confluence of the McNamara fallacy, the target culture, managerialism, political and media opportunism, and common-or-garden unkindness. Jarman's HSMR was widely and erroneously believed to measure 'avoidable' deaths in hospitals; that is, deaths directly caused by poor care. The Stafford scandal led to several official inquiries, including two by Sir Robert Francis QC. There was a further inquiry in 2013 by the NHS's medical director, Professor Sir Bruce Keogh, into fourteen other hospitals with a high HSMR. The story of Sir Brian Jarman and his HSMR is a stark warning on how metrics mislead medicine.

Jarman worked initially as a GP in London, but moved into academe and was appointed professor of primary health care at St Mary's Hospital in 1984, and later head of the division of primary care at Imperial College. He became an eminent member of the British medical establishment: he was knighted in 1998, and elected president of the British Medical Association in 2003. Jarman was keen on statistics and health informatics and developed socio-economic indicators such as the Underprivileged Area Score, or Jarman Index. In the early 1990s, he turned his attention to hospital mortality rates, and developed the Hospital Standardized Mortality Ratio (HSMR). The formula for the Hospital Standardized Mortality Ratio is: HSMR = (Actual deaths/expected deaths) x 100. An HSMR of 100 therefore means the actual death rate was the same as the expected death rate. The cause of death was taken from the discharge 'codes': after the death of a patient, a hospital clerk – a 'coding officer' – goes through the notes and allocates a specific code for the main or primary diagnosis, and also codes for other diagnoses, or 'co-morbidities'. These numerical codes are based on the international classification of disease (ICD). This coding is not always accurate, being subject to the clarity of the clinical notes and the vigilance of the coding officer. The health informatics expert Paul Taylor explained how the HSMR is determined:

Data on actual deaths were taken from HES [Hospital Episode Statistics] and restricted to in-hospital deaths. A logistic regression model was used to calculate the risk of death for the 50 most common diagnoses, which account for over 80 per cent of admissions, based on a set of factors: sex, age, admission method (non-elective or elective), socio-economic deprivation quintile of the area of residence of the patient, diagnosis/procedure sub-group, co-morbidities, number of previous emergency admissions, year of discharge, month of admission and the source of admission, and the use of the ICD code for palliative care. Using data on the mix of these factors seen by each trust, they calculated the expected death rate.

In 1999, Jarman joined the panel of the Kennedy Inquiry into the children's heart surgery unit at Bristol Royal Infirmary. The scandal was a turning point in the history of the NHS: British medicine would never be quite the same. It started when Steve Bolsin, an anaesthetist at the hospital, expressed concern about the high mortality rate among babies and children undergoing cardiac surgery. The media reported a simplistic narrative of incompetent surgeons presiding over a blood-bath of dead babies. The truth was both more com-plicated and banal: the surgeons took on cases they should have sent elsewhere, and the cardiac surgery unit was under-staffed and underfunded. One of the key recommendations of the Kennedy Inquiry was that hospital mortality rates should be made more widely available. In the same year that Jarman joined the Bristol Inquiry, he and his colleagues at Imperial published a paper in the *British Medical Journal* entitled 'Explaining differences in English hospital death rates using routinely collected data'. Coming out in the middle of the Bristol scandal, this was hot stuff. This paper outlined the HSMR statistical methodology, and reported variations in mortality rates across hospitals in England. The paper had a political message, showing a strong link between hospital death rates and the ratios of doctors (both in hospitals and general practice) to number of population served. Jarman wrote to the secretary of state for health, Frank Dobson, asking if he could publish the HSMRs of various English hospitals; Dobson refused. In September 2000, Jarman met with two journalists, Tim Kelsey of the *Sunday Times* and Roger Taylor of the *Financial Times*. They had both covered the Bristol story, and saw an unexploited commercial potential in Jarman's HSMR. Kelsey and Taylor co-founded Dr Foster Intelligence (DFI), whose first *Good Hospital Guide* appeared in 2001. DFI was established as a commercial enterprise, which would earn its income from the *Good Hospital Guide* (which published HSMRs and hospital league tables) and by selling its services to hospital trusts. It claims: 'We are the leading provider of healthcare variation analysis and clinical benchmarking solutions worldwide.' The former health secretary Alan Milburn was an enthusiastic supporter, and hospitals were told to collaborate with DFI whether they liked it or not. Milburn's successor, Patricia Hewitt, bought the company in 2006 for £12m; this deal went through without a competitive tender. Roger Taylor is still director of research at Dr Foster, and describes himself as an 'entrepreneur, journalist and author'

– 'statistician' is conspicuously absent from this list. Tim Kelsey is now CEO of the Australian Digital Health Agency. Taylor and Kelsey must be very grateful indeed to Jarman for giving them such a commercial opportunity. Confusingly, maddeningly and bizarrely, the academic unit that Jarman led at Imperial College was named the Doctor Foster Unit (DFU). Jarman has always claimed that the Doctor Foster *Unit* is completely independent of Dr Foster *Intelligence*: he admitted, however, to the second Francis Inquiry that 47 per cent of DFU's funding came from DFI.

In 2007, DFI's *Good Hospital Guide* gave the Mid Staffordshire NHS Trust an HSMR of 127, the fourth highest in the country. The trust thought that inaccurate coding might be the cause of the high HSMR: a review of case notes led to recoding in several cases. The trust also commissioned two epidemiologists from Birmingham University, Professor Richard Lilford and Dr M. A. Mohammed, to examine the statistical methods used to calculate the HSMR. Lilford and Mohammed were known critics of the HSMR; they argued that it was susceptible to all sorts of biases, such as the accuracy of coding, local GP care, the proportion of admissions that are emergency, and local access to hospice beds. They concluded that this method could not possibly measure 'avoidable' deaths, and thus the quality of care. Many other statisticians and health informatics experts agreed with them. Stafford Hospital and its HSMR might have remained a local or, at least, regional concern had it not been for a woman called Julie Bailey. Her eighty-six-year-old mother, Bella, died at the hospital on 8 November 2007, after being admitted eight weeks earlier with 'an inflamed hiatus hernia'. The Bailey family was shocked by the poor nursing care at the hospital. Bailey complained to the hospital CEO Martin Yeates, but received no response. She wrote a letter to the local newspaper and was contacted by several other families who had similar experiences; the response prompted Bailey to set up a local pressure group called 'Cure the NHS'. This group, consisting of local people whose relatives had died at Stafford Hospital, held its first meeting in December 2007 at Breaks, the café run by Bailey.

Meanwhile, the Healthcare Commission, aware of the high HSMR at Stafford Hospital, carried out an investigation between March and October 2008; the report was published in March 2009. The Commission was not impressed by the hospital's explanation for the high HSMR – namely, that it was primarily due to poor coding. Details of the report were leaked to the press before publication. Among these details was an estimated 400 to 1,200 excess (and by extrapolation 'avoidable') deaths over a period of more than a decade. These figures did not appear in the final, published report, but were leaked to the press, who put these numbers in their headlines; they are, to this day, still presented as evidence. When the Commission's report was published, Prime Minister Gordon Brown and Health Secretary Alan Johnson apologized to the patients and families who had experienced poor care at the hospital. CEO Martin Yeates was suspended and the chairman Toni Brisby resigned. Alan Johnson was replaced by Andy Burnham on 5 June 2009, and on 21 July 2009, he announced that there would be a further, independent inquiry into Stafford Hospital, which would be chaired by Robert Francis QC. The report of this Inquiry was published on the 24 February 2010.

The Inquiry devoted much time to mortality rates at the hospital, and Francis relied greatly on Jarman's evidence. The report contains the now-famous table of the HSMRs at Stafford Hospital from 1996 to 2008, with the final figure of an excess of 1,197 'observed' over 'expected' deaths. Francis expressed doubts about the HSMR statistics, pointing out that later figures for Mid Staffordshire showed 'an astonishing apparent recovery': the HSMR for 2008/9 was down to 89.6, and in the *Good Hospital Guide 2009*, Stafford was one of the top 14 hospitals. While acknowledging Sir Brian Jarman's reputation and eminence, Francis suggested that statistics such as the HSMR should be produced by an independent government-funded agency, not by a commercial enterprise such as DFI. Jarman, however, was careful to point out to the Inquiry that all 'excess' deaths were not necessarily 'avoidable':

We recognize that mortality alerts and HSMRs cannot be used as a direct tool for discovering failings in hospitals... What the data does... is pose the question:

what is the explanation for your high mortality for the particular diagnosis or procedure that has alerted that month? We make it very clear in the alert letter that we send to Trusts that we draw no conclusions as to what lies behind the figures.

Francis finally ruled that no conclusions could be drawn from the HSMR figures:

Taking account of the range of opinion offered to the Inquiry, including a report from two independent experts, it has been concluded that it would be unsafe to infer from the figures that there was any particular number or range of numbers of avoidable or unnecessary deaths at the Trust.

The story, and Robert Francis, didn't end there. In June 2010, the new (Conservative) Health Secretary Andrew Lansley announced that there would be another public inquiry, which would again be chaired by Francis. Cure the NHS had complained that the first Inquiry was not public, and Francis himself thought its remit too narrow. Francis reopened for business in November 2010, and another report was published in February 2013. Yet again, he heard evidence from Sir Brian, but Jarman, by this stage, seems to have tested even Francis's patience: 'The Inquiry received voluminous and detailed evidence and analyses from Professor Jarman.'

Francis 2 covered much the same territory as Francis 1, such as the by now infamous table 'provided by Professor Brian Jarman' on HSMRs at Stafford from 1996 to 2009. Professor Sir Bruce Keogh expressed major concerns about the HSMR:

Potentially 'avoidable' deaths cannot be identified *a priori*, with the result that there can be no 'gold standard' against which to assess the sensitivity and specificity of purely statistical measures such as HSMRs; and that no single measure can possibly encapsulate all aspects of the quality of care offered by a hospital... I have major reservations with the presentation of simplistic 'league tables' of HSMRs.

Ian Kennedy also criticized the HSMR: 'Professor Sir Ian Kennedy told the Inquiry that, at the time, the HSMR was not widely accepted as predicting risk or underperformance.' Francis clearly did not enjoy the protracted haggling over the HSMR methodology; the report is littered with phrases such as 'to the non-statistician' and 'if I understand correctly'. He concluded, somewhat wearily, much as he had after the first Inquiry, that 'to this day, there is no generally accepted means of producing comparative figures, and unjustifiable conclusions continue to be drawn from the numbers of deaths at hospitals and about the number of avoidable deaths'. The media and politicians must have skimmed through Francis's report of 783,710 words; they maintained their belief that there had been 1,200 'avoidable' deaths at Stafford. The *Guardian* was the only newspaper which later admitted – in 2015 – that this figure was entirely bogus, and that its own reporting of the numbers had been incorrect.

Stafford Hospital was probably no worse, and no better, than many other NHS district general hospitals. Many local people deeply resented Julie Bailey's campaign; she received anonymous hate mail, and her mother's grave was vandalized. She left Stafford in 2013, several months after the publication of the second Francis Report. Stafford, like many hospitals, struggled with poor morale, inadequate staffing and facilities, the pressure of targets and the ever-increasing demands of an ageing and frailer population. The witness statements made for harrowing reading, but was Stafford really a rotten apple, an outlier? I witnessed, during the fourteen years I worked in the NHS, episodes of cruelty and neglect as bad as those described at Stafford, in hospitals that were regarded as 'centres of excellence'. What happened at Stafford and what happened, and still happens, in many other NHS hospitals was the result of a toxic combination of decades of managerialist totalitarianism, understaffing and the steady decline in the professional standards of doctors and nurses. Robert Francis, the eminent and sweetly reasonable silk, didn't understand that acute medical wards are constantly on the edge of chaos, understaffed and leaderless; that most beds are occupied by highly dependent elderly patients; that senior and experienced nurses have abandoned these wards for easier roles; that form-filling and box-ticking have been prioritized over patient care. His two inquiries were triggered by bogus statistics, but Francis seemed to find it difficult to believe that the method which produced these statistics could be produced by a man as eminent as Professor Sir Brian Jarman.

Less than three weeks before the publication of Francis 2, Sir Bruce Keogh announced that he would be conducting a review of urgent and emergency care in the NHS, focusing particularly on fourteen hospitals, like Stafford, with a high HSMR. His report was published in July 2013. He wrote to Jeremy Hunt, secretary of state for health: 'However tempting it may be, it is clinically meaningless and academically reckless to use such statistical measures [as the HSMR] to quantify actual numbers of avoidable deaths.' Keogh told Hunt where the real problems lay: 'Some hospital trusts are operating in geographical and academic isolation... the lack of value and support being given to frontline clinicians, particularly junior nurses and doctors... the imbalance that exists around the use of transparency for the purpose of accountability and blame rather than support and improvement.' Keogh also commissioned a review into the relationship between the HSMR and 'avoidable' deaths, which was carried out by Nick Black (professor of health services research) and Lord Ara Darzi. Their review was published in the *British Medical Journal* in 2015. They randomly selected 100 deaths from 34 trusts, and found that the proportion of avoidable deaths was low (3.6 per cent), with no significant association with HSMRs. A similar (if smaller) external review of deaths at Stafford Hospital – commissioned by the Mid Staffordshire NHS Foundation Trust – had been carried out by Dr Mike Laker (of Newcastle University) in 2009. He reviewed 120 case notes and interviewed 50 families. He concluded that poor care had led directly to death in 'perhaps one'.

The letter from Keogh to Hunt was written on 16 July 2013. Two days earlier, the *Sunday Telegraph* published an article called 'Labour's "denial machine" over hospital death rates':

> Professor Sir Brian Jarman, of Imperial College London, worked on a government review which will this week show that 14 hospital trusts have been responsible for up to 13,000 'excess deaths' since 2005.
>
> … Prof Sir Bruce Keogh will describe how each hospital let its patients down badly through poor care, medical errors and failures of management, and will show that the scandal of Stafford Hospital, where up to 1,200 patients died needlessly, was not a one-off.

The media clearly loved Jarman; here is a 2014 profile by the *Guardian*: 'Ever ready to take a journalist's phone call and with a pithy quote for every occasion, the eighty-year-old remains a reporter's friend. He is also a spiky proponent of his brainchild: the hospital standardized mortality ratio

(HSMR).' A month after the publication of the Keogh report, Sir David Spiegelhalter wrote a commentary in the *British Medical Journal*. Spiegelhalter is a distinguished statistician: Winton professor for the public understanding of risk at Cambridge University, fellow of the Royal Society and president of the Royal Statistical Society. He examined the media outrage over hospital deaths:

> So where did the '13,000' come from? It is the difference between the observed and 'expected' number of deaths in the 14 trusts between 2005 and 2012. The *Telegraph* claims this number is based on research by Professor Brian Jarman, one of the Keogh team, and the numbers can be derived from data on the HSMR available on Jarman's website. It should have been fairly predictable that such a briefing to journalists would be misleadingly reported... we would expect at any time that around half of all trusts would have 'higher than expected' mortality, just by chance variability around an average... The difference between the observed and expected number of deaths has been called 'excess deaths', a term used in the Bristol Royal Infirmary Inquiry: as head of that statistical team, I deeply regret this use as it so readily translates, whether through ignorance or mendacity, into 'needless deaths'... Like the '1,200' at Mid Staffs, '13,000' threatens to become a 'zombie statistic' – one that will not die in spite of repeated demolition.

Spiegelhalter's contrition over his clumsy use of the term 'excess deaths' at Bristol is telling. Professor Sir Brian Jarman, however, is not given to such expressions of public contrition, and was undaunted by the thrashing of his statistical baby by Sir Bruce Keogh and many others. If anything, it stiffened his resolve. In September 2017, the *Mail on Sunday* carried a piece entitled: 'NHS buries 19,000 "suspect" deaths: expert demands urgent probe into "avoidable" fatalities amid shock claims dozens of hospitals across Britain are "potentially unsafe"':

> Professor Sir Brian Jarman says his shocking findings mean there are dozens of 'potentially unsafe' hospitals that should be investigated over high death rates, but which are being overlooked... He calculated that there were 32,810 'unexpected' deaths in English hospitals over the past five years. But using the NHS's preferred method, only 13,627 were classed as such – a difference of 19,183 deaths.

Jarman's prominent status in the British medical establishment has given him a public platform from which he terrifies the general public through his regular briefing of journalists. Francis indulged him and stopped short of direct criticism only because he is so eminent. It is too late for Jarman to admit that he was wrong: he has invested his entire career and academic credibility in the HSMR.

Robert McNamara, however, was big enough to admit in his old age that he had been wrong. During his long post-White House career, he repeatedly revisited his Vietnam experience to see what could be learned from it. At the age of eighty-five, he told an interviewer: 'I'm at an age where I can look back and derive some conclusions about my actions. My rule has been: Try to learn. Try to understand what happened. Develop the lessons and pass them on.' He devoted his later years to doing just that. He met with the North Vietnamese general Vo Nguyen Giap, and learned that the US had failed to understand their adversary: 'We saw Vietnam as an element of the Cold War, not what they saw it as, a civil war.' McNamara admitted that this failure 'reflected our profound ignorance of the history, culture and politics of the people in the area and the personalities and habits of their leaders'. When he died in 2009, the *Economist* observed: 'He was haunted by the thought that amid all the objective-setting and evaluating, the careful counting and the cost-benefit analysis, stood ordinary human beings. They behaved unpredictably.'

McNamara's career is also a great example of the cult of managerialism which came to dominate, in the second half of the twentieth century, not just business, but also many other spheres of human activity, including health care, education and government. McNamara was a great exemplar of the new manager: 'A trained specialist in the science of business management who is also a generalist moving easily from one technical area to another.' Writing in the *Harvard Business*

Review in 1980, Robert H. Hayes and William J. Abernethy blamed managerialism (at least in part) for America's economic decline:

> What has developed, in the business community as in academia, is a preoccupation with a false and shallow concept of the professional manager, a 'pseudoprofessional' really – an individual having no special expertise in any particular industry or technology who nevertheless can step into an unfamiliar company and run it successfully through strict application of financial controls, portfolio concepts, and a market-driven strategy.

The obsession with metrics in medicine is partly due to managerialism. The delusion that generic business methods can be easily applied to the complexities of health care has been perpetuated by famous managerialists such as Sir Gerry Robinson. Less than two weeks after the publication of the second Francis report, he wrote an opinion piece for the *Daily Telegraph* entitled: 'Yes, we can fix the NHS':

> Imagine a McDonald's in Leicester, say, where things are going wrong. Perhaps the wrong number of chicken nuggets are being handed out, or the washrooms aren't supplied with soap. These problems would show up immediately via a weekly reporting system which compared its performance against every other McDonald's

in the country, and you'd have a senior manager down in days to sort out the problems.

To the metrics-driven managerialist, running the NHS is essentially no different from ensuring a uniformity of customer experience at the many McDonald's outlets.

The target culture was partly to blame for Stafford. To meet financial targets to become a foundation trust, the hospital sacked 150 staff and closed 100 beds (18 per cent of the total). The hospital had one of the lowest numbers of ward nurses in the country, with a deficit of 120 nursing posts. The Healthcare Commission Inquiry found that junior doctors were routinely diverted from duties on the general wards and redeployed to the emergency department, so the hospital would not be in breach of the four-hour target (the target for patients attending emergency departments to be seen, treated, and either admitted or discharged). This left the general wards unstaffed and dangerous. The politicians who expressed their shock and outrage over Stafford were often the very same ministers who had imposed these targets. Although John Major's Conservative government started the process in the early 1990s with the Patient's Charter, it was the Blair administration which really embraced targets. These targets initially focused on such matters as waiting times, cleanliness and average length of hospital stay. Ian Blunt, health services analyst at the Nuffield Trust, wrote: 'One of the fundamental challenges to targets is that they measure what can be counted rather than what matters. This is particularly true when a target (one tiny slice of activity) is used to infer quality (which is the result of a complex array of care processes and interactions).' Blunt noted that, when first introduced, NHS targets were generally achieved because of increased funding and central support. Targets, however, came with an inevitable and predictable downside: 'Methods such as increasing the risk of managers being sacked and public "naming and shaming" led to dysfunctional behaviour such as "gaming" data, short-termism, bullying and obsessive checking and assurance activities.' Targets can work if used sparingly in a few well-chosen areas, and backed up with additional resources. If more targets are added willy-nilly, they create a climate of confusion in hospitals about their priorities. Targets, which were intended to guide and promote good care, have become an end in themselves, often leading to a grotesque inversion of their original purpose.

NHS consultants are familiar with stories of patients having major operations cancelled so the target for elective surgery for patients with minor ailments can be met. Most will be familiar, too, with the cynical, and sometimes bizarre, ruses employed by managers to meet the four-hour emergency department target. The Academy of Medical Royal Colleges and Faculties in Scotland spoke for many in the NHS with their 2015 document *Building a More Sustainable NHS in Scotland*: 'The current approach to setting and reporting on national targets and measures, while having initially delivered some real improvements, is now creating an unsustainable culture that pervades the NHS. It is often skewing clinical priorities, wasting resources and focusing energy on too many of the wrong things.' Even the politicians – traditionally the great supporters of NHS targets – are beginning to have reservations. The Scottish Conservatives expressed these doubts in their manifesto for the 2016 general election ('A world-class health-care system for your loved ones'): 'We want our doctors making the best medical decision for a successful outcome, rather than feeling they have to service the input targets.' Less than a year later, however, in February 2017, the same Scottish Conservatives attacked the Scottish National Party government for its failure to reach outpatient waiting list targets.

In 2015, Dr Foster Intelligence published a report called *Uses and Abuses of Performance Data in Healthcare*. Roger Taylor, co-founder of DFI, was one of three authors, none of whom has a professional qualification in statistics or epidemiology. When a body such as Dr Foster, whose entire *raison d'être* is health-care metrics, publishes a paper detailing the limitations of such metrics, one should sit up and take notice. They clearly saw no irony in producing a document criticizing the metrics obsession that was directly behind their own foundation. The document listed the unintended adverse consequences of targets as: (1) tunnel vision: focusing on aspects of clinical performance that are measured and neglecting unmeasured areas; (2) inequity – for example, surgeons may avoid operating on the most seriously ill patients because they fear a 'poor outcome' with such patients may drive up their individual mortality rates; (3) bullying; (4) erosion – diminution of professional motivation; (5) ceiling effect – removing incentives for further improvement; (6) gaming; and (7) distraction – challenging, obfuscating or denying data which suggest underperformance. DFI suggested several steps to 'reduce data abuse', such as improving the quality of data and considering the potential for gaming. The heart surgeon Professor Stephen Westaby wrote a piece for the *Spectator* which showed how publishing cardiac surgeons' death rates led to 'adverse selection':

> Mortality rates were published hastily. Surgeons were 'named and shamed' – a phrase destined to become enshrined in NHS folklore. Very rapidly the emphasis shifted from patient care to self-preservation. So many people contribute to the recovery of a heart surgery patient that the simplest way to stay under the radar is to avoid the sickest patients. Low risk translates into low mortality.

Why do such 'pseudoprofessionals' as Roger Taylor, Joanne Shaw and Katy Dix wield more influence over health policy than the likes of Stephen Westaby? The contemporary distrust of 'experts' is partly to blame. Since the Thatcher reforms in the late 1980s, the NHS has provided rich pickings for management consultants and other opportunists keen to 'exploit the commercial potential' of whatever fad is grabbing the politicians' attention. Modern politicians are more comfortable in the company of businessmen, management consultants and journalists than they are with professors of surgery and fellows of the Royal Society. They know that after leaving office, they may well be working with these same businessmen, journalists and management consultants. The phenomenon of the 'revolving door' between ministerial office and the private sector is now accepted as the way of the world: after Alan Milburn (so keen on Dr Foster Intelligence) resigned as health secretary in 2003, he took up a consultancy post with Bridgepoint Capital, a venture capital firm which funds private finance initiatives for the NHS. The politicians and journalists who expressed their shock and outrage over Stafford have moved on, as they always do, and Stafford Hospital must somehow keep going, its name forever sullied and tainted, bound for eternity to the corpses of the zombie stories and the zombie statistics.

It would be foolish to argue that metrics have no place in medicine, but over-emphasis on such metrics has distracted contemporary medicine from its true purpose. Numbers should be our tool, not our tyrant. Society's main concern about medicine is lack of compassion. This concern, as the Stafford scandal showed, is justified, and many doctors and nurses see this as the greatest challenge for contemporary health care. The components of compassion – kindness, courage, competence, bottom – are unquantifiable. The 'invisible glue' – the goodwill which once held together organizations like the NHS – has vanished.

13

THE MENDACITY OF EMPATHY

The mortality figures at Stafford distracted attention from what was most shocking about the story: the culture of neglect and cruelty at the hospital. The witness statements to the first Francis Inquiry described an institution bereft of common human decency, where sick elderly people were left to lie in their own excrement. The scandal led to a predictable reaction from the medical establishment, with a slew of statements from the royal colleges asking what could be learned from Stafford? Many – especially those positioned well away from the wards and the emergency departments – declared that the real problem was a lack of empathy. There are currently over 1,500 books listed on Amazon with 'empathy' in the title. From government to health care to education, empathy is the putative fix for all our societal woes. Some commentators, such as Peter Bazalgette, author of *The Empathy Instinct* (2017), proposed that NHS doctors and nurses should undergo formal empathy training. Such training is now embedded in US medical training, because empathy is now one of the accredited skills required by the American Council for Graduate Education in Medicine. Empathy is thus doing a brisk trade in the big business (and new member of the medical–industrial complex) that is medical education, and the journals regularly feature earnest articles on how to teach it. A systematic review published in 2014 in the journal *BMC Medical Education* identified over 1,400 papers on empathy. One study 'sought to build medical student empathy for patients receiving injections by asking medical students to take turns injecting each other with saline solution'. Others used 'role playing' and 'reflective writing'. Although the authors of this review were keen to promote these toe-curling endeavours, they conceded that 'the majority of studies lacked highly rigorous designs'.

Big Science is muscling in, too. Empathy is the latest target of the neuroscience based on functional magnetic resonance imaging (fMRI) of the brain. 'Functional' MRI differs from standard MRI scanning by mapping the differential rate of oxygen consumption in specific parts of the brain; this is thought to measure metabolic, and hence neuronal, activity. Functional MRI scans display impressive colour changes which reflect these differences in oxygen consumption: if an area of the brain 'lights up' during a specific activity, it is assumed that this activity 'takes place' in that location. The sociologist Scott Vrecko listed fMRI-based neurobiological accounts of altruism, borderline personality disorder, criminal behaviour, decision-making, fear, gut feelings, hope, impulsivity, judgement, love, motivation, neuroticism, problem gambling, racial bias, suicide, trust, violence, wisdom and zeal. Many commentators have called this branch of neuroscience the contemporary equivalent of phrenology, the bizarre belief – which had a remarkable hold on the public imagination in the nineteenth century – that personality and intellectual ability could be determined by examination of the contours of the skull. Phrenology eventually died out, mainly because it had no plausible scientific basis, and because it was used to give a bogus scientific credibility to racism. The neo-phrenology based on fMRI has been called 'neurobollocks' by its detractors. It has infiltrated economics, criminology, theology, literary criticism, education, sociology and politics; the American writer Matthew Crawford described fMRI as 'a fast-acting solvent of critical faculties'. Some more cautious scientists, however, are painfully aware of its limitations; the neuroscientist David Poeppel observed that 'we still don't understand how the brain recognizes something as basic as a straight line'. Functional MRI scanning is also a contributor to the Replication Crisis in Big Science, as exemplified by the notorious 'dead salmon' study. The academic psychologist Craig Bennett of the University of California Santa Barbara was concerned about 'random noise' causing spurious false-positive results from fMRI scanning. To investigate this 'random noise', he purchased a (dead) salmon from a fish-monger and carried out a series of fMRI scans. Having been placed in the scanner, 'the salmon was shown a series of photographs depicting human individuals in social situations with a specific emotional valence'. The salmon was scanned and 'several active voxels were discovered in a cluster located within the salmon's brain cavity'. (The three-dimensional image produced by fMRI is built up in units called 'voxels': each voxel represents a tiny cube of brain tissue.)

As well as the obligatory fMRI-based neuroanatomy, all contemporary meditations on empathy contain earnest accounts of mirror neurons, described as 'the most hyped concept in neuroscience'. These cells were first described in the 1990s by the Italian neuroscientist Giacomo Rizzolatti, who studied macaque monkeys, and noticed that the monkeys' 'pleasure centres' were activated by the sight of seeing a human engaged in a pleasurable activity (eating peanuts). He also found that some motor cells (involved in the control of movement) are activated by the sight of the same movement in others (humans and monkeys). Since then, outlandish claims have been made for these neurons, particularly by the Indian-American neuroscientist V. S. Ramachandran, who believes these cells are responsible for empathy, language, even civilization. A sobering review of mirror neurons by the British neuroscientists James Kilner and Roger Lemon, published in *Current Biology* in 2013, concluded that we can't extrapolate findings in monkeys to humans; we're not absolutely sure if these cells exist in humans; and even if they do, we're not sure what their function is. These doubts haven't remotely impeded the establishment of the new popular science orthodoxy which holds that mirror neurons are what make us human and empathetic. Neurobollocks has escaped from the laboratory and is now the rickety foundation for popular, and populist, books by writers such as Jonah Lehrer, Malcolm Gladwell and many others. Writing in the *New Statesman* in 2012, Steven Poole described this phenomenon as 'an intellectual pestilence' and observed how putting the prefix 'neuro' to whatever you are talking about gives it a pseudo-scientific respectability.

Several recent books give us breathless accounts of the neuroscience of empathy. Here is a passage from Peter Bazalgette's *The Empathy Instinct*:

> In 1994, [Simon] Baron-Cohen identified another region of the empathy circuit – the *orbitofrontal cortex*... And in 2013, Tania Singer and colleagues at the Max Planck Institute in Germany hit on another piece of the jigsaw. The *right supramarginal gyrus* helps us to separate our own feelings about a situation from those of the subject of our empathy.

Bazalgette's sketchy understanding of how scientific inquiry works doesn't inhibit him in the least, and he concludes that therapeutic applications of this neuroanatomical knowledge

239

are just around the corner: 'Routine fMRI scans will identify psychopaths and others with an empathy deficit as people requiring special attention. There will be programs to repair the parts of their brains which malfunction.' He suggests that 'there is an argument for the screening of all of those in the front line of patient care. This would require the development of new emotional intelligence and empathy tests.' In the near future, he seems to suggest, would-be doctors will undergo fMRI scanning of their orbitofrontal cortex and right supra-marginal gyrus.

Dr Helen Riess is a psychiatrist at Harvard Medical School and is an expert in teaching empathy. Having first developed a shaky, unpersuasive scaffolding of neuroscience (the standard stuff about fMRI and mirror neurons) around empathy training, she then set up a for-profit company called Empathetics™ which offers empathy training for medical students, nurses and doctors. (The word 'empathetics' gives the impression that this is a new branch of medicine, sounding, as it does, vaguely like 'anaesthetics'.) Riess has even produced a study showing that doctors who had been through her course were rated by patients as being 'more empathetic': a good example of the new trend for advertising disguising itself as 'research'. 'Empathetics' is closely related to another American medical movement called 'Narrative Medicine', whose high priestess is Dr Rita Charon of Columbia University. It is no coincidence that both Narrative Medicine and Empathetics took root and flourished in the US, where the dominant ethos in medicine is consumerism. Doctors can indeed be trained to simulate the outward expressions of empathy – maintaining eye-contact, giving the 'correct' verbal prompts, and so on. This is similar to acting; indeed, out-of-work actors often find employment as 'patients' in such exercises. The title essay of Leslie Jamison's 2014 collection *The Empathy Exams* recounts her experience as a medical actor, a 'standardized patient' for the training of medical students. These 'patients' have to give an evaluation of the students' performance:

> Checklist item 31 is generally acknowledged as the most important category: 'Voiced empathy for my situation/problem'. We are instructed about the importance of this first word, *voiced*. It's not enough for someone to have a sympathetic manner or use a caring tone of voice. The students have to say the right words to get credit for compassion.

Jamison observed that some students cynically game this po-faced charade: 'I grow accustomed to comments that feel aggressive in their formulaic insistence.' Although her writing is characterized by a relentless and wearisome solipsism, Jamison has a moment of insight when she began to obsessively check her face for weakness after her brother developed Bell's palsy (facial paralysis): 'I wonder if my empathy has always been this, in every case: just a bout of hypothetical self-pity projected onto someone else.'

The new discipline of medical humanities also claims to develop empathy in medical students and doctors. It began in the 1970s with modest aims, covering such ground as ethics and the history of medicine. It turned its attention to great works of literature with the hope that these books could teach something about the experience of illness and the business of doctoring. So, for example, Tolstoy's novella *The Death of Ivan Ilyich* is often used to teach students about what Dame Cicely Saunders called 'total pain', meaning the kind of extreme existential suffering experienced by some dying people. Some students thought it useful, others didn't. In the early years, courses in medical humanities were generally taught by doctors who happened to have an interest in literature, history and ethics, but the discipline was gradually annexed by professional humanities academics, chiefly because it attracted significant funding from bodies like the Wellcome Trust. (Yet another example of how easily medicine is colonized by rival professions who have spotted an opportunity.) The medical schools weren't aware of the seismic changes in the humanities that began in the 1960s. Doctors and medical students were mystified by post-modernist claims that there was no objective truth, that all written documents – including scientific papers – were 'narratives', informed by the cultural and economic milieu of the authors. Post-modernism's high priests – such as Foucault and Derrida – were also aggressively anti-science. These academics brought to the subject this post-modernist world view, and an incomprehensible jargon.

Here is a typical sentence from a 2011 article in the journal *Medical Humanities* entitled 'Medical humanities as expressive of Western culture': 'The act of asserting disciplinarity, even interdisciplinarity, derives momentum from a certain teleological impetus to self-narrate, producing a coherent or centralizing version of self-hood in relations to one's envisaged audience.' This passage is reminiscent of the infamous 1996 Sokal hoax, when the eminent physicist Alan Sokal submitted a paper to the American journal *Social Text* entitled 'Transgressing the boundaries: towards a transformative hermeneutics of quantum gravity'. The paper, a deliberate parody of post-modernist gobbledygook, was accepted and published. The new journals devoted to the medical humanities can only be read – and are only meant to be read – by a small, highly specialized, academic audience. I looked through a recent issue of the journal *BMJ Medical Humanities*, and found words like assemblage, hybridity, concorporeality, durative, anthropogony, postconventional, embodied (selves and materialities), and, of course, 'narrative'. The jargon of the medical humanities bears a striking resemblance to that of conceptual art, so mocked by the cultural critic Jonathan Meades: 'It is the language of the trained liar, of the professionally mendacious... impenetrable to the uninitiated, a language of exclusion.'

Narrative Medicine, with its glutinous mix of virtue signalling, pseudo-biblical language and social justice agenda, is the dominant and unchallenged orthodoxy within the medical humanities. Robin Downie lamented the obsession with 'narrative' and pointed out that doctors have always listened to the patient's story – it was called taking a history. The Narrative Medicine lobby believes that patients are ill served by a medical establishment that is relentlessly mechanistic and dehumanizing. 'Inevitably', wrote the doctor and philosopher Raymond Tallis in *Hippocratic Oaths* (2004) 'many commentators trained in the humanities, and remote from the responsibility for making and acting on correct diagnoses, see the tussle or tension between stories as a hermeneutic power struggle, with the omnipotent doctor crushing the powerless patient with his version of events.' Some students question, not unreasonably, what these cloistered academics can possibly teach them about the challenges of medical life and dealing with the sick and dying. A group of students from four English medical schools wrote a short piece for the journal *Clinical Teacher* entitled 'Hold my hand while you misdiagnose me', arguing that the curriculum in medical schools had become over-concerned with 'soft' skills at the expense of medical knowledge.

The soft skill most touted is 'communication'. Many educators – particularly those who never have to deal with real patients – sincerely believe that they can teach it. Those who actually practise medicine are not quite so convinced. Addressing the British Psychological Society in 1955, Richard Asher trashed this notion, one of the articles of faith most cherished by that particular audience:

the way we deal with our patients, and especially how we talk to them, is about the most important part of our trade; but can it be taught? I doubt it. It can be learned by experience and to some extent by watching great doctors handling their patients, but it cannot be taught like pharmacology. All the power of tongue and pen, and all the wisdom of textbook and lecture can never teach a doctor the knowledge of when to probe, when to speak and when to keep silent. They are private mysteries with a different solution for every one of the million permutations of personality involved between a doctor and his patient.

Jane Macnaughton argued, in a much-cited 2009 *Lancet* essay, that empathy is neither desirable nor teachable:

it is potentially dangerous and certainly unrealistic to suggest that we can really feel what someone else is feeling. It is dangerous because, outside the literary context, where we are allowed direct experience of what a fictional patient is feeling, we cannot gain direct access to what is going on in our patient's head... a doctor who responds to a patient's distress with 'I understand how you feel' is likely, therefore, to be both resented by the patient and self-deceiving.

Empathy can clash with other moral considerations and

sways us towards the needs of the few over the many. We see this phenomenon in health-care spending. Empathy and awareness raising are closely related, and equally mendacious. Writing in the *Irish Times*, the health economist Anthony McDonnell took the example of the Irish government's decision to fund the cystic fibrosis drug Orkambi, which costs €100,000 to treat a single patient for a year. Cystic Fibrosis Ireland is a powerful advocacy group, and many patients with the disease are articulate and media-savvy: 'At a time when our health system is struggling to stay afloat we should refocus the resources we have, where they can achieve the most good for the greatest number of people possible, rather than cherry-picking people on how sad their story appears.'

Compassion and empathy are often used interchangeably, but they are entirely different qualities. One can be empathetic without being compassionate: psychopaths and bullies, for example, tend to be very skilled in divining people's emotions. Similarly, one can be compassionate without being particularly empathetic, as good doctors often are. Empathy can be a hindrance to doctors in their work, as over-identification with the patient's distress might distract the doctor from *doing* something to relieve that distress. Older, more stoically inclined patients value other qualities such as competence, honesty and respect. Paul Bloom interviewed a surgeon for his polemical book *Against Empathy* (2016):

Christine Montross, a surgeon weighs in on the risks of empathy: 'If, while listening to the grieving mother's raw and unbearable description of her son's body in the morgue, I were to imagine my own son in his place, I would be incapacitated. My ability to attend to my patient's psychiatric needs would be derailed by my own devastating sorrow. Similarly, if I were brought in by ambulance to the trauma bay of my local emergency department and required immediate surgery to save my life, I would not want the trauma surgeon on call to pause to empathize with my pain and suffering.'

Dr Joel Salinas's memoir, *Mirror Touch: Notes from a Doctor Who Can Feel Your Pain* (2017), is presented as the confession of a super-empathizer, but is an unintentionally comic warning of the dangers of empathy for a doctor. Salinas is a young (mid-thirties) Boston-based neurologist, who claims to suffer from a condition called 'polysynesthesia'. Chromo-synaesthesia – where some people experience sounds as colours – is well recognized. Salinas, however, has multiple forms of synaesthesia, including 'mirror-touch' synaesthesia, which causes him to *feel* the pain others experience. In Wes Anderson's film, *The Royal Tenenbaums*, the neurologist and author Raleigh St Clair (played by Bill Murray and based on Oliver Sacks) studies a pre-adolescent boy called Dudley Heinsbergen, who has a rare neurological syndrome characterized by 'amnesia, dyslexia and colour blindness, with an acute sense of hearing'. St Clair exhibits Dudley at medical schools and hospitals, and writes a bestselling book called *Dudley's World*. Joel Salinas is the Dudley Heinsbergen of empathy. His memoir has all the key components of the contemporary medical quest memoir: 'I knew at an early age I was different, even though I didn't know how or why I was different… I remember asking my mother why no one seemed to like me.' He visits the laboratory of V. S. Ramachandran in San Diego (he of mirror neurons fame), and after a battery of psychometric tests is told he has 'mirror-touch synesthesia'. He travels to London to attend a meeting of the UK Synaesthesia Association, and takes the opportunity to visit the laboratory of the neuroscientist Michael Banissey at University College London, where he has a further round of tests, which confirm the diagnosis.

You would think that medicine would be an eccentric career choice for a polysynaesthete, yet he enrols at the University of Miami Medical School. He spends some time in Gujarat in India, where he gets his first exposure to obstetrics, which doesn't go well: 'As I watched the obstetricians perform an episiotomy, slicing their surgical scissors across a woman's flesh, I felt my pelvic diaphragm stretching and nearly shred… I felt desecrated. I felt powerless. Yet no one seemed to notice or care, not even the woman who had just given birth.' (I mused here that a woman who had just given birth after an episiotomy might have more on her mind than a queasy medical student.) During his first week as an internal medicine resident, he is called to a cardiac arrest: 'The sensations in my body mirrored the sensations in his. Compression after compression on his chest and on mine.' The book is crammed with these experiences: when a patient is undergoing a lumbar puncture (spinal tap), Salinas feels the needle going into his own back; when a trauma patient undergoes an abdominal surgical exploration, he feels the knife going in; dealing with a manic patient, he become manic too: 'I had the physical sensation, as if I had just drunk several shots of espresso'. Salinas can even empathize with death:

> Whenever a patient died, I felt as if I had died, too. The feeling never waned. In this regard, I have died many times. Watching patients pass away, I realized in my body the final moments before fading into death... Like Lazarus, I stand regularly at the threshold and behold an altar with enough space for a new sense of the divine...

He found himself 'gravitating towards the study of empathy', and assures us that 'the mirror neuron system is a generally accepted theory about how the brain works'. Were Raleigh St Clair to write *Joel's World*, he might describe Salinas's syndrome as a rare neurological condition characterized by solipsism, humbug and relentless self-promotion. Salinas, in his modish, up-to-the-minute feel for the zeitgeist, is in his own way as odious as the legendary bullies who dominated

British medicine in the 1950s and 1960s. When I started in the profession, medicine accommodated such bullies; now it provides a home for swooning empaths.

In the decade since the Stafford Hospital scandal began, the NHS has been regularly accused of an institutional lack of compassion. Stafford, however, was nothing new, and was not an isolated case. The story of inhumane and cruel treatment of patients at Ely Hospital in Wales broke in 1967; an inquiry by Geoffrey Howe was published in 1969. Between Ely and Stafford there were several official inquiries into poor care at various NHS hospitals. The ranks of doctors and nurses have always contained a minority of the lazy and the unkind. We delude ourselves if we believe that this minority can be identified and weeded out at recruitment. What did change between Ely and Stafford, however, was the unintended, unforeseen and perverse disincentivization of compassion. The target culture has created many new unintended consequences and perverse incentives, skewing clinical priorities and distracting staff from providing compassionate care. Metrics have become more important than patients. Many senior experienced ward nurses now view this work as intolerable and are leaving their posts for less stressful positions as specialist nurses and managers: there is no incentive – professional or financial – for them to stay on the wards. This has created a vacuum where leadership is most needed.

Sir David Weatherall, regius professor of medicine in

Oxford, wrote an essay for the *British Medical Journal* in 1994, called 'The inhumanity of medicine', in which he drew attention to this professional and institutional disincentivization of compassion: 'From the time that they [doctors] decide on a career in medicine until they retire, many of them live in such an overcharged atmosphere, and one in which the demands on them are now so great, that sometimes the central reason for what they are doing – that is, the wellbeing of their patients – is forgotten.' What can be done about this? 'Legge's Axioms' might guide us. Sir Thomas Legge (1863–1932) was the first medical inspector of factories in Britain. He is famous for his four axioms on the prevention of occupational lead poisoning, which appeared in his posthumously published book, *Industrial Maladies*. The first two axioms are: (1) 'Unless and until the employer has done everything – and everything means a good deal – the workman can do next to nothing to protect himself although he is naturally willing enough to do his bit', and (2) 'If you can bring an influence external to the workman, you will be successful; if you can't, or don't, you won't.' In other words, institutional and organizational change is far more likely to succeed than attempts to change the behaviour of individuals. Compassion will not be regenerated by educational workshops, or by increasing even more the already stifling regulation of doctors and nurses; if anything, this only exacerbates the problem. The average doctor and nurse is, to use Legge's phrase, 'naturally willing enough to do his bit'. We should instead remove the institutional and organizational perverse incentives which act as barriers to compassionate care.

Empathy is easy, and useless, serving only the desire of the empath to feel good about themselves, and to announce their virtue. Medicine needs compassion, not empathy. Compassion is not easy, because it is composed of more than simple human kindness. Compassion also requires courage, competence and bottom. Compassion means that not only do you recognize suffering and distress, you *do* something to relieve it. Empathetics™ and the Narrative Medicine Program at Columbia may be able to teach medical students and doctors glib customer skills and a superficial carapace of 'caringness', but the regeneration of compassion in our hospitals will require a more fundamental shift in the culture of contemporary health care.

14

THE MIRAGE OF PROGRESS

Progress – rather than compassion – is the core belief of the medical–industrial complex. The philosopher John Gray wrote that 'questioning the idea of progress at the start of the twenty-first century is a bit like casting doubt on the existence of the Deity in Victorian times'. The belief in progress reflects the power of science to change our lives. Over the last one hundred years, longevity has increased dramatically, and immunization has reduced or eradicated diseases that used to kill millions of people. The benefits of science seem so self-evident that only a fool or a madman would question it, or the idea of progress. But science, which gave us all these unalloyed benefits, also gave us nuclear bombs and napalm; it is entirely possible that technology may render the world uninhabitable for humans. Then, progress will end. John Gray has never denied the reality of scientific progress, or its benefits, but has consistently argued that although scientific knowledge increases from generation to generation, gains in ethics and politics are more easily lost: 'They have to be learned afresh with each new generation.'

Every new 'advance' in medicine is a genie that cannot be put back in the bottle. Big Science isn't going to suddenly become thoughtful, scholarly Little Science. Pharma isn't going to develop a social conscience in late middle age. The medical misinformation mess is now a foetid swamp that may never be drained. As once-poor countries develop and become richer, they develop Western appetites for all sorts of commodities, particularly medicine. End of life care among wealthy Indians, for example, now brings them the worst excesses of American medicine. At present, medical 'progress' gives us the dubious and ruinously expensive gift of helping us to survive long enough to experience loss of independence and chronic disease. We must surely have better, nobler ambitions than to survive into a frail old age. We are not a mere *homo economicus*, or the bundle of diagnoses that is *homo infirmus*. Medicine is the bully that is stealing from education, from decent affordable housing, from the arts, from good public transport. Our ever-increasing spending on it is not giving us any greater comfort or joy.

We need a reformed medicine, but how is that going to happen? Too many have a vested interest in unreformed medicine continuing, so it is very unlikely to happen by a societal consensus; we will have to be forced into doing it.

What would force us? The most likely events are economic collapse and a global pandemic of a new, untreatable infectious disease on a background of climate change and exhaustion of the earth's resources by globalization. In such a scenario, medicine would have to shrink down to treating the victims of this pandemic and providing basic measures such as immunization, trauma care and obstetrics. This scenario is not as unlikely as you might imagine. Martin Rees, the astronomer royal, predicted in his 2003 book *Our Final Century* that 'the odds are no better than fifty-fifty that our present civilization... will survive to the end of the present century... unless all nations adopt low-risk and sustainable policies based on present technology'. The Stockholm Resilience Centre, a research institute for sustainability and environmental issues, has defined nine boundaries that must be maintained to ensure a flourishing civilization. Five of these boundaries have been crossed: extinction rates, climate change, phosphorous and nitrogen cycles, land-use change and ocean acidification. Tom Koch, an expert in emerging diseases, reckons that in less than a decade we will have a major pandemic of a new infectious disease; one that will be untreatable, which will affect 60 per cent of the world's population, and will kill 30–35 per cent of those infected.

Microbiologists have been warning for some years that resistance to antibiotics is steadily rising: what was once a concern is now a crisis. The problem was predicted as far back as 1945 by the discoverer of penicillin, Sir Alexander Fleming: 'The public will demand [the drug], and then will begin an era of abuses.' New antibiotic development has stalled, mainly because these drugs are not profitable enough for the pharmaceutical industry. Pharma is interested mainly in blockbuster drugs (such as statins) that are used for decades, not in antibiotics that are given for a week. The Office of Health Economics in London estimated that the net present value of a new antibiotic is only about $50 million, while a drug used to treat a chronic neuromuscular disease is worth $1 billion. Compared with new cancer drugs, antibiotics are simply too cheap for Big Pharma to bother with. Meanwhile, overuse of the antibiotics we currently have may lead to most of them becoming useless, with the consequences of routine surgery becoming impossible and sepsis untreatable. Para-doxically, sepsis awareness campaigns, which contribute sub-stantially to overuse of antibiotics, may create a future when sepsis is untreatable.

The achievements of medicine's golden age are astonish-ing, a one-off in human history – a unique confluence of events, science and chance. Since then, the production of data has risen exponentially; the yard is covered with bricks, but the edifice is no nearer completion and, if anything, is crumbling. The quarter-trillion dollars spent annually on medical research is mainly wasted, and simply fills the yard with bricks that will never be used to build anything. Mean-while, people get old, get sick and die, as they always did.

Even if progress continued at the rate of the mid-twentieth century, it would probably not be in our best interest, with an ever-diminishing young generation supporting millions of centenarians. What would happen if we won the War on Cancer and could reverse dementia? What would we die of then? Would 'old age' become, again, an acceptable 'cause of death' on a death certificate? Would that modern fairy tale, the 'compression of morbidity', finally come true? This concept, first elaborated by the Stanford medical professor James Fries in 1980, claims that as longevity steadily rises, old age will be a time of increasingly prolonged good health, with an ever-shorter period of illness prior to death. American baby-boomers, bombarded with images of marathon-running centenarians, have invested heavily in this fairy tale, and are desperate for it to be true. Unfortunately, it isn't. In a 2010 review of trends in mortality and disability in the US, Eileen Crimmins and Hiram Beltrán-Sánchez, from the Davis School of Gerontology at the University of Southern California, concluded: 'The compression of morbidity is a compelling idea. People aspire to live out their lives in good health and to die a good death without suffering, disease, and loss of function. However, compression of morbidity may be as illusory as immortality. We do not appear to be moving to a world where we die without experiencing disease, functioning loss, and disability.'

René Dubos (1901–82), the French-American microbiologist, environmentalist and writer, wrote *Mirage of Health*

(1959) more than twenty years before James Fries came up with the idea of the compression of morbidity, and observed that this fantasy has been with us since antiquity:

> In *Works and Days* Hesiod wrote of the golden age when men 'feasted gaily, undarkened by sufferings' and 'died as if falling asleep'. The oldest known medical treatise written in the Chinese language also refers to the health of the happy past. 'In Ancient times,' states the Yellow Emperor in his *Classic of Internal Medicine* published in the fourth century BC, 'people lived to a hundred years, and yet remained active and did not become decrepit in their activities.'

The Marquis de Condorcet (1743–94), the Enlightenment figure most associated with the new religion of progress, predicted a future in which 'man would be free from disease and old age and death would be indefinitely postponed'. Several books were written in the late eighteenth century on this theme, such as *The Art of Prolonging Life* by C. W. Hufeland and Johann Peter Frank's *A Complete System of Medical Policy*. The Enlightenment, having banished religious superstition, created a new belief – and a new form of enslavement – that the human body is a machine, governed by mechanistic and deterministic laws. *Mirage of Health* appeared at the peak of medicine's golden age. Dubos, indeed, had contributed significantly to one of the great achievements of the golden age – the development of antibiotics. In the very first page, Dubos cast doubt on the great project of which he was a part:

> Complete freedom from disease and from struggle is almost incompatible with the process of living... The very process of living is a continual interplay between the individual and his environment, often taking the form of a struggle resulting in injury or disease... Complete and lasting freedom from disease is but a dream remembered from imaginings of a Garden of Eden designed for the welfare of man... it is easier for the scientific mind to unleash natural forces than for the human soul to exercise wisdom and generosity in the use of power... solving problems of disease is not the same thing as creating health and happiness.

Dubos argued, as did others – most notably Thomas McKeown – that the great improvements in public health and longevity happened long before the golden age of medical research and was achieved by better sanitation and nutrition. He wittily observed how medicine took credit for these gains: 'When the tide is receding from the beach it is easy to have the illusion that one can empty the ocean by removing water with a pail.'

Mankind has always yearned for utopias, but only in our age did this yearning become medicalized. The World Health Organization (WHO) was established immediately after the war in 1946, and in its constitution defined health as 'not merely the absence of disease or infirmity, but a state of complete physical, mental and social wellbeing'. Petr Skrabanek joked that ordinary people might achieve this sort of feeling 'fleetingly, during orgasm, or when high on drugs'. In 1975, the director-general of the WHO, Dr Halfdan Mahler (a Dane) gave an address to the organization entitled 'Health for All by the Year 2000!' This ludicrous slogan was adopted by the WHO as a mission statement for the 1970s and 1980s, but the millennium came and went without Mahler's utopia. He wasn't alone: in 1987, the eminent Irish cardiologist Professor Risteard Mulcahy told the *Irish Times*: 'By the year 2000 the commonest killers such as coronary heart disease, stroke, respiratory disease and many cancers will be wiped out.' Many people in rich countries began to believe the WHO's definition of health, and when they found themselves experiencing the inevitable hardships of human life, and thus temporarily not in a state of 'complete physical, mental and social wellbeing', presented themselves to doctors so that they might be restored to the blissful state promised by the WHO as the birthright of all humans. This intolerance of distress is partly to blame for the exponential rise in the prescribing of antidepressant and anxiolytic drugs. The criteria now used by GPs to diagnose depression are now so flimsy that a combination of two weeks' unhappiness accompanied by other symptoms such as insomnia is enough to diagnose a 'major depressive episode': up to 50 per cent of the population may experience such an event over a lifetime.

Meanwhile, those with severe, persistent depression – what used to be called melancholia – struggle to access psychiatric services. The vast increase in diagnosis of attention deficit hyperactivity disorder (ADHD), autism and bipolar disorder cannot be accounted for by an increase in prevalence. Neither religion nor philosophy claims that life should be happy, but the WHO does.

The ancient Greeks had two separate, rival and distinct medical traditions, those of Aesclepius and Hygieia. The Aesclepian tradition, which the late GP Ian Tate called the 'for God's sake do something' school, has come to dominate medicine. This model concentrated on the specific causes of disease, whereas the Hygieian tradition emphasized health as being in harmony with oneself and the environment. Hygieians recommended correct living and taking responsibility for one's health, while Aesclepians went to doctors instead: 'While Asclepius is in Luther's words only "God's body patcher",' wrote Dubos, 'the serene loveliness of Hygieia in the Greek marble symbolizes man's lofty hope that he can someday achieve a state of harmony within himself and with the surrounding world.' Aesclepian thinking led to the concept of a 'magic bullet' for every disease. René Dubos called this Aesclepian formulation of disease 'the doctrine of specific aetiology': 'By equating disease with the effect of a precise cause – microbial invader, biochemical lesion, or mental stress – the doctrine of specific aetiology had appeared to negate the philosophical view of health as equilibrium and to render obsolete the traditional art of medicine.' The doctrine of specific aetiology stands on some shaky scientific foundations. Tuberculosis, for example, is assumed to be 'caused' by the tubercle bacillus, yet many millions carry this organism and never develop the disease of tuberculosis. The bacillus generally requires the assistance of poverty and malnutrition. *Helicobacter pylori* similarly 'causes' duodenal ulcer, yet the vast majority of people infected with the bacterium will never develop a duodenal ulcer, a disease that was in steep decline long before *Helicobacter* was identified as the 'cause'. This Aesclepian thinking may also account for the failure, so far, of Big Science, the new genetics and precision medicine to deliver the kind of advances predicted of them. 'Despite its obvious limitations,' observed Richard Smith, 'the magic bullet model seems alive and well in the age of genetics and personalized medicine. Pharmaceutical companies are merchants of magic bullets and keen to keep the fantasy alive. It's also very attractive to the public, which can fantasize that a pill will fix their problems.' Humans, and human diseases, are infinitely more complex than we imagine, a truth which the great cancer biologist Robert Weinberg was humble enough to admit to. We may have already achieved most of the medical advances we are ever going to achieve, and in some areas – such as antibiotic resistance – we are going backwards. Many have argued that if we simply applied uniformly, equitably and rationally all the scientific knowledge we currently possess

– that which we *already know* – medicine and health would be transformed.

People have always been enchanted by the prospect of miracles. As faith in God and gods has waned, we look to science. Both René Dubos and Ivan Illich argued that medicine had taken over the role of religion in the Western world; we now expect the partnership of medicine and the state to oversee our health. Dubos observed that this pact came at a cost:

> But too often the goal of the planners is a universal grey state of health corresponding to absence of disease rather than to a positive attribute conducive to joyful and creative living. This kind of health will not rule out and may even generate another form of ill, the boredom which is the penalty of a formula of life where nothing is left unforeseen.

Medicine is now ruled by a very feeble philosophy that sees man as a machine, concerned only with material comfort and survival into extreme old age. This philosophy, as René Dubos observed, might be applied to ants and cows, but not to humans. We are made to struggle, to embrace dangers. We value some things beyond mere comfort: 'The satisfactions which men crave most and the sufferings which scar their lives most deeply, have determinants which do not all reside in the flesh or in the reasonable faculties and are not completely accounted for by scientific laws.' Our faith in progress, and that science will deliver it, perpetuates the illusion that we can plan our society to maximize health and happiness. This faith is, in the unlikely phrase of Bertrand Russell, a form of cosmic impiety. We know we have despoiled the environment, and suspect we may pay a heavy price. We know that human life, art, religion, spirituality and love are based on the eternal verities of growing old and dying, yet we now subscribe to the notion that we should struggle against these verities. It is a struggle that we are not winning, that we cannot win, and that we shouldn't win. Ivan Illich took from Greek mythology the example of the brothers Prometheus and Epimetheus. Prometheus stole fire from the gods, and for his hubris suffered the eternal punishment of having his liver pecked out every day by an eagle (and also the indignity of being used as an illustration by liver specialists for every lecture on the remarkable capacity of that organ to regenerate itself). Epimetheus allowed Pandora to open her box of plagues, but held on to hope. Illich called for 'the Rebirth of Epimethean Man', whose guiding spirit is hope, rather than the Promethean spirit of expectation. Epimethean Man stands in a humble, creaturely relationship to nature and his creator. Promethean Man, with his institutions, regulations and predictions, expects to control his destiny and conquer nature.

Medicine no longer knows what it is *for*. Is the ultimate aim of medical research to eliminate all disease? If so, then it must be aiming, too, to make us immortal. Even if that were possible (which it isn't), are we quite sure that we want it? Is the aim of clinical medicine now to keep the entire adult population under permanent surveillance by screening for an increasing number of diseases? Does longevity trump all other considerations? Medicine, and particularly medical research, operates in an economic and moral vacuum, choosing to ignore the societal implications of cancer treatments and 'precision medicine' which give tiny, incremental gains at huge cost. We embrace the advantages of globalization, but not the duties. We in the rich West cannot continue to spend vast sums for such modest gains while people die in poor countries of diseases that can be cheaply cured and prevented. They also die without adequate pain relief or palliative care: the *Lancet* Commission on Alleviating the Access Abyss in Palliative Care and Pain Relief (2017) described how '61 million are affected by severe health-related suffering, 80 per cent of whom live in low and middle-income settings. 45 per cent of those dying annually experience severe suffering, including 2.5 million children.' Richard Horton, the editor of the *Lancet*, wrote an extraordinary editorial (which could have passed as the work of Ivan Illich) in which he laid the blame for this 'sea of suffering' on the medical–industrial complex:

> Medicine regards the alleviation of suffering as someone else's problem. Palliative care is too often seen to indicate failure – the failure of medicine to cure. The hubris

of modern medicine is that it cannot face up to failure. The deification of biomedicine as a discipline dedicated exclusively to survival has created an anti-humanist and quasi-theocratic science of health.

Some, such as Richard Smith, have argued that we should concentrate on getting treatments that work to those who currently have no access to them, rather than developing new highly expensive treatments which only increase inequality. Julian Tudor Hart (1927–2018), a GP who campaigned against health inequality, coined the phrase the 'Inverse Care Law' in 1971: 'The availability of good medical care tends to vary inversely with the need for it in the population served.' North America, for example, has 2 per cent of the health burden, but 25 per cent of the health-care workers, while Africa has 25 per cent of the burden and 2 per cent of the workforce. In the twenty-first century, the main determinants of health are income and living environment, not medicine.

The trench war will eventually end, through either sheer exhaustion or the collapse of the civilization that sustains it. Ronald Wright, in his book *A Short History of Progress*, described how various civilizations throughout history (Sumer, Rome, the Maya) collapsed, mainly because they destroyed the environment that had supported them. Polynesians settled on Easter Island around the eighth century AD. Ancestor worship was the main religious observance of these settlers, and each clan constructed stone images to honour their fore-fathers. The construction of these images required large quantities of wood, rope and manpower, and the statues grew ever larger. The island's trees were being hewn down faster than they could be replaced by growth, and eventually the land was desolate, leading to wars over the scarce resources and a collapse in population: 'The people had been seduced by a kind of progress that becomes a mania, an "ideological pathology", as some anthropologists call it. When Europeans arrived in the eighteenth century, the worst was over; they found only one or two living souls per statue, a sorry rem-nant, "small, lean, timid and miserable", in Cook's words.' The statue cult of Easter Island was an ideological pathology. Medicine's Aesclepian/Cartesian quest to abolish or prevent all disease is an equally self-destructive mania. It may also be proved irrelevant far sooner than we think. Our overcrowded, hyperconnected world is an ideal incubation environment for new infectious diseases, against which our current anti-microbial drugs may be impotent. The anthropologist and historian Joseph Tainter warned that 'collapse, if and when it comes again, will this time be global... World civilization will disintegrate as a whole.'

The great medical statistician Major Greenwood was pro-fessor of epidemiology at the London School of Hygiene and Tropical Medicine from 1929 to 1945, and mentor to Austin Bradford Hill. In a speech to the Royal Society of Arts in 1931, he laid out the ethos of the school: 'The ambition of the school should be to become the spiritual home of men and women, differing in race, education and practical ambitions, but all aspiring to do their part to make the conditions of human life everywhere more bearable.' Greenwood's humble aspiration is rather moving. He did not promise to 'cure all disease', or 'defeat cancer'. Perhaps contemporary medicine should embrace as its mission 'to make the conditions of human life everywhere more bearable'. That is what medicine is for.

EPILOGUE

During the golden age, medical science gained huge prestige, and human life and death became medicalized. Despite its global dominance, the medical–industrial complex has given us meagre, feeble comforts at vast expense. Its chief concern is its own survival and continued dominance, and its ethos now is a betrayal of the scientific ideals of the golden age. Clinical practice, too, has become a vast industry, concerned mainly with degenerative disease and old age, and the herding of entire populations – through screening, awareness raising, disease mongering and preventive prescribing – into patient-hood.

Patients are increasingly unhappy with medicine. This is because they expect too much of it, and because only people of my mother's age remember what being sick was like before the golden age. Doctors are just as unhappy. They know, deep down, that their powers are limited, yet ever more responsibilities and demands are laid at their door. Hospitals have become clearing houses for old people; normal variations in human behaviour and emotion are now the object of phar-maceutical intervention; life's inevitable existential problems are brought to the doctor to solve. What can we do? Medi-cine has become a pseudo-religion; our patients must be gently encouraged into apostasy and renunciation. George Bernard Shaw advised his readers to use up their health, and not to outlive themselves. We might similarly encourage our patients to lead what James McCormick called lives of modi-fied hedonism, 'so that they might enjoy to the full the only lives that they are likely to have, rather than to portray life as a journey beset with avoidable dangers'. We might admit to ourselves that we have over-valued our knowledge, and over-promised to our patients. We might admit, too, that the war against death is unwinnable, and refocus our energies instead on an equitable sharing of what we already know and have, and towards a new medicine that values healing and the relief of suffering.

The current priorities of medicine – with the cathedral-like teaching hospitals and biomedical research at the top, and community and hospice care at the bottom – will have to be turned upside down. I am not optimistic that this will happen. Strong societal forces will almost certainly ensure that the current consensus prevails. These forces include the commodification of all human life, the over-weening power of giant international corporations, the decline of both politics and the professions, the sclerosis of compliance and regulation, the fetishization of safety, the narcissism of the Internet and social media, but above all the spiritual dwarfism of our age, which would reduce us to digitized machines in need of constant surveillance and maintenance. The medical–industrial complex is not some vast, organized, sentient conspiracy; it is as fallible, messy and irrational as the people who created it. It has become so powerful, however, that medicine has now passed the Illichian tipping point where it is doing more harm than good to the people it is supposed to serve. There are two simple questions to ask of any new development, treatment or paradigm in medicine: first, who benefits? *Cui bono*? And second, does it make life any sweeter? Ask these questions of genomics, digital health and awareness campaigns, and the answers are obvious.

Temperamentally, I was made for the cloister, for the library, but fate placed me in the dust of the arena. *Aoibhinn beatha an scoláire* ('how sweet is the scholar's life!'), wrote an anonymous seventeenth-century Irish poet. I sometimes speculate on what a life of the mind might have been like, but this is idle. I have lived instead in a world of pain, sickness and death, but also in a world of intimacy, humour and life. I look forward to being relieved soon of the sometimes unbearable burden of responsibility. My younger colleagues are as seduced by new fads and fallacies as I was at their age, but pointing this out to them would be sour and ungracious. It took more than three decades for me to figure out what was going on around me, and to realize that medicine – clinical medicine, that is – is a difficult career for a sceptic. Never-theless, rational scepticism is as necessary to the practice of medicine as compassion: doctors need to be both Humean and humane. As I near the end of this career, I find it not exactly easier, but less difficult. I no longer worry about litigation and protocols, and talk to my patients as I would to a friend or a relative: honestly, as doctors should. I have been pleasantly surprised that they seem to find this candour a release, as it gives them the opportunity to talk about what really matters. Both we and our patients have been enslaved by the medical–industrial complex, and it is time we rebelled. Society needs to reach a new accommodation with old age and death. Doctors need to proclaim that professionalism and clinical judgement are still – and will always be – the core of what we do. We need to stop hiding behind protocols, edicts and fear of sanction, and simply try to make the conditions of human life more bearable. Orthodoxies in science and practice come and go, but the core of doctoring stays the same. We may not be able to cure, but we can still heal.

My younger self would, I think, approve of my late apos-tasy. I like to think, too, that the shades of Ivan Illich, his disciple John Bradshaw, the Czech contrarian Petr Skrabanek and that scourge of lazy thinking Richard Asher are in some way appeased.

ACKNOWLEDGEMENTS

My editor Neil Belton gave me unfailing encouragement and much valuable advice. Thanks also to Florence Hare at Head of Zeus, and to my agent Jonathan Williams. I have previously written on some of the themes of this book for the Dublin Review of Books and the Journal of the Royal College of Physicians of Edinburgh: thanks to Maurice Earls and Enda O'Doherty at the *DRB* and to Rona Gloag, Allan Beveridge and Martyn Bracewell at the *JRCPE*. I thank John Wilson, who introduced me to the McNamara fallacy, and Eugene Cassidy, with whom I had an illuminating conversation about contemporary psychiatry. Richard Smith's blogs, tweets, emails and conversations have been consistently inspiring. I am grateful to my colleagues – Orla Crosbie, Syed Akbar Zulquernain and Clifford Kiat – who have supported me in many practical ways. Thanks, as always, to Karen, James and Helena.

BIBLIOGRAPHY

Academy of Medical Sciences (2015) 'Reproducibility and reliability of biomedical research: improving research practice'. Online at https://acmedsci.ac.uk/viewFile/56314e40aac61.pdf

Academy of Medical Royal Colleges and Faculties in Scotland (2015) *Building a More Sustainable NHS in Scotland: Health Professions Lead the Call for Action.*

Adams, Stephen and Martyn Halle (2017) 'NHS buries 19,000 "suspect" deaths: expert demands urgent probe into "avoidable" fatalities amid shock claims dozens of hospitals across Britain are "potentially unsafe"'. *Mail Online*, 2 September. Online at www.dailymail.co.uk/news/article-4847184/Expert-demands-urgent-probe-avoidable-fatalities.html

Adams, Tim (2013) 'Mid Staffs whistleblower Julie Bailey: "I don't go out here on my own any more"'. *Guardian*, 27 October. Online at www.theguardian.com/society/2013/oct/27/julie-bailey-mid-staffordshire-nhs-whistleblower

Aggarwal, Ajay, T. Fojo, C. Chamberlain, C. Davis and R.

Sullivan (2017) 'Do patient access schemes for high-cost cancer drugs deliver value for society? Lessons from the NHS Cancer Drugs Fund'. *Annals of Oncology* 28:1738–50.

Ajana, Btihaj (2017) 'Digital health and the biopolitics of the Quantified Self'. *Digital Health* 3:1–18.

Alexander-Williams, John and Jeremy Hugh Baron (1987) 'British Society of Gastroenterology 1937–87: an overview'. *Gut* 28:S53–5.

Altman, Douglas (1994) 'The scandal of poor medical research'. *British Medical Journal* 308:283–4.

Anderson, C.M., J.M. French, H.G. Sammins, A.C. Frazer, J.W. Gerrard and J.M. Smellie (1952) 'Coeliac disease: gastrointestinal studies and the effect of dietary wheat flour'. *Lancet* 1:836–42.

Angell, Marcia (2000) 'Is academic medicine for sale?' *New England Journal of Medicine* 342:1516–18.

Annan, Noel (1990) *Our Age: Portrait of a Generation*. London: Weidenfeld & Nicolson.

Apolone, G., R. Joppi, V. Bertele and S. Garattini (2005) 'Ten years of marketing approvals of cancer drugs in Europe'. *British Journal of Cancer* 93:504–9.

Arie, Sophie (2017) 'Simon Wessely: "Every time we have a mental health awareness week my spirits sink"'. *British Medical Journal* 358:j4305.

Arrow, Kenneth (1963) 'Uncertainty and the welfare economics of medical care'. *The American Economic Review* LIII(5): 141–9.

Asher, Richard (1949) 'The seven sins of medicine'. *Lancet* 2(6574): 358–60.

—(1951) 'Munchausen's Syndrome'. *Lancet* i:339–41.

—(1954) 'Straight and crooked thinking in medicine'. *British Medical Journal* 2(4885):460–2.

—(1955) 'Talk, tact and treatment'. *Lancet* 268:758–60.

—(1961) 'Apriority: thoughts on treatment'. *Lancet* 2(7217): 1403–4.

—(1972) *Talking Sense*. London: Pitman Medical.

—(1984) *A Sense of Asher: A New Miscellany*. Ed. Ruth Holland. London: British Medical Association.

Avery Jones, Francis (1943) 'Haematemesis and melaena: with special reference to bleeding peptic ulcers'. *British Medical Journal* 2:689–91.

Ball, Madeleine P., Jason R. Bobe, Michael F. Chou, Tom Clegg, Preston W. Estep, Jeantine T. Lunshof, Ward Vandewege, Alexander Wait Zaranek and George M. Church (2014) 'Harvard Personal Genome Project: lessons from participatory public research'. *Genome Medicine*, 6:10. Online at https://genomemedicine.biomedcentral.com/track/pdf/10.1186/gm527

Bastian, Hilda (2006) 'Down and almost out in Scotland: George Orwell, tuberculosis and getting streptomycin in 1948'. *Journal of the Royal Society of Medicine* 99:95–8.

Bazalgette, Peter (2017) *The Empathy Instinct: How to Create a More Civil Society*. London: John Murray.

BBC News (2007) 'Friends fund Wilson's cancer drug'. *BBC*

News, 11 July. Online at http://news.bbc.co.uk/2/hi/uk_news/
england/manchester/6293176.stm

Bennett, Craig M., Abigail A. Baird, Michael B. Miller and George
L. Wolford (2009) 'Neural correlates of interspecies perspective taking in the post-mortem Atlantic Salmon: an argument for multiple comparisons correction'. Online at http://
www.prefrontal.org/files/posters/Bennett-Salmon-2009.pdf

Bevan, A. (1951) *Democratic Values. First in the Series of Fabian
Autumn Lectures 1950: Whither Socialism? Values in a Changing Civilization*. London: Fabian Publications.

Biagioli, Mario (2016) 'Watch out for cheats in citation game'.
Nature 535:201.

Biesiekierski, Jessica R., Simone L. Peters, Evan D. Newnham,
Ouriana Rosella, Jane G. Muir and Peter R. Gibson (2013)
'No effects of gluten in patients with self-reported non-celiac
gluten sensitivity after dietary reduction of fermentable,
poorly absorbed, short-chain carbohydrates'. *Gastroenterology* 145:320–8.

Black, J. W., W. A. M. Duncan, C. J. Durant, C. R. Ganellin and
E. M. Parsons (1972) 'Definition and antagonism of histamine H_2-receptors'. *Nature* 236:385–90.

Black, Nick (2010) 'Assessing the quality of hospitals'. *British
Medical Journal* 340:c2066.

Bloom, Paul (2016) *Against Empathy: The Case for Rational
Compassion*. London: The Bodley Head.

Blunt, Ian (2015) *Fact or Fiction? Targets Improve Quality in
the NHS?* Nuffield Trust comment, 13 February. Online at

www.nuffieldtrust.org.uk/news-item/fact-or-fiction-targets-improve-quality-in-the-nhs

Boodman, Sandra G. (2017) 'The other big drug problem: older people taking too many pills'. *Washington Post*, 9 December. Online at https://www.washingtonpost.com/national/health-science/the-other-big-drug-problem-older-people-taking-too-many-pills/2017/12/08/3cea5ca2-c30a-11e7-afe9-4f60b5a6c4a0_story.html?noredirect=on&utm_term=.5c2fa76c8f43

Booth, Christopher C. (1997) 'Factors influencing the development of gastroenterology in Britain'. In *Gastroenterology in Britain: Historical Essays*. Ed. W.F. Bynum. London: Wellcome Trust.

Booth, Christopher M. and Elizabeth A. Eisenhauer (2012) 'Progression-free survival: meaningful or simply measurable?' *Journal of Clinical Oncology* 30:1030–3.

Boseley, Sarah (2017) 'Cancer Drugs Fund condemned as expensive and ineffective'. *Guardian*, 28 April. Online at https://www.theguardian.com/science/2017/apr/28/cancer-drugs-fund-condemned-as-expensive-and-ineffective

Bowman, Andrew (2012) 'The flip side to Bill Gates' charity billions'. *New Internationalist*, 1 April. Online at https://newint.org/features/2012/04/01/bill-gates-charitable-giving-ethics

Bradshaw, John (1978) *Doctors on Trial*. London: Wildwood House.

Breathnach, C.S. and J.B. Moynihan (2011) 'William Wilde and the early records of consumption in Ireland'. *Ulster Medical Journal* 80(1):42–8.

British Society of Gastroenterology (1987) *British Society of Gastroenterology 1937–1987: A Selection of Scientific Papers.* London: Smith Kline & French Laboratories.

Brooks, David (2013) 'The philosophy of data'. *New York Times*, 4 February. Online at https://www.nytimes.com/2013/02/05/opinion/brooks-the-philosophy-of-data.html

Brouns, Fred J. P. H., Vincent J. van Buul and Peter R. Shewry (2013) 'Does wheat make us fat and sick?' *Journal of Cereal Science* 58:209–15.

Browne, Noël (1986) *Against the Tide.* Dublin: Gill & Macmillan.

Buckley, Martin J. M. and Colm A. O'Morain (1998) '*Helico-bacter* biology – discovery'. *British Medical Bulletin* 54:7–16.

Buranyi, Stephen (2017) 'The hi-tech war on science fraud'. *Guardian*, 1 February. Online at www.theguardian.com/science/2017/feb/01/high-tech-war-on-science

—(2017) 'Is the staggeringly profitable business of scientific publishing bad for science?' *Guardian*, 27 June. Online at www.theguardian.com/science/2017/jun/27/profitable-business-scientific-publishing-bad-for-science

Burnet, Sir Macfarlane (1971) *Genes, Dreams and Realities.* New York: Basic Books.

Bush, Vannevar (1945) *Science: The Endless Frontier. A Report to the President on a Program for Postwar Scientific Research.* Washington, DC: National Science Foundation.

Bynum, Bill (2008) 'The McKeown thesis'. *Lancet* 371:644–5.

Callahan, Daniel and Sherwin B. Nuland (2011) 'The quagmire: How American medicine is destroying itself'. *New Republic*, 19 May. Online at https://newrepublic.com/article/88631/american-medicine-health-care-costs

Campbell, Donald T. (1979) 'Assessing the impact of planned social change'. *Evaluation and Program Planning* 2(1):67–90.

Carbone, David P., Martin Reck, Luis Paz-Ares, Benjamin Creelan *et al.* (2017) 'First-line Nivolumab in stage IV or recurrent non-small-cell lung cancer'. *New England Journal of Medicine* 376:2415–26.

Carreyrou, John (2018) *Bad Blood: Secrets and Lies in a Silicon Valley Startup.* New York: Alfred A. Knopf.

Catassi, Carlo (2015) 'Gluten sensitivity'. *Annals of Nutrition and Metabolism* 67(suppl 2):16–26.

Catassi, Carlo, Luca Elli, Bruno Bonaz, A. *et al.* (2015) 'Diagnosis of non-celiac gluten sensitivity (NCGS): the Salerno experts' criteria'. *Nutrients* 7:4966–77.

Chalmers, I., M. Enkin and M.J.N.C. Keirse (1989) *Effective Care in Pregnancy and Childbirth.* Oxford: Oxford University Press.

Chalmers, Iain (2008) 'Archie Cochrane (1909–1988)'. *Journal of the Royal Society of Medicine* 101:41–4.

Chalmers, Iain and Paul Glasziou (2009) 'Avoidable waste in the production and reporting of research evidence'. *Lancet* 374:86–9.

Charlton, Bruce G. (2009) 'Why are modern scientists so dull? How science selects for perseverance and sociability at the expense of intelligence and creativity'. *Medical Hypotheses* 72(3):237–43.

—(2012) *Not Even Trying: The Corruption of Real Science.* Buckingham: University of Buckingham Press.

Charon, Rita (2001) 'Narrative medicine: a model for empathy, reflection, profession, and trust'. *Journal of the American Medical Association* 286:1897–902.

Chief Medical Officer for Scotland Annual Report 2014–15 (2016) *Realistic Medicine.* Online at http://www.gov.scot/Publications/2016/01/3745

Clark, Jocalyn and Linsey McGoey (2016) 'The black box warning on philanthrocapitalism'. *Lancet* 388:2457–8.

Clifford, Clark (with R. Holbrooke) (1991) *Counsel to the President: A Memoir.* New York: Random House.

Clinical Evidence (2015) 'What conclusions has Clinical Evidence drawn about what works, what doesn't based on randomised controlled trial evidence?' Online at https://bestpractice.bmj.com/info/evidence-information

Cochrane, Archibald L. (1972) *Effectiveness and Efficiency: Random Reflections on Health Services.* London: The Nuffield Provincial Hospitals Trust.

Cockburn, Patrick (2005) *The Broken Boy.* London: Jonathan Cape.

Coghlan, J.G., D. Gilligan, H. Humphries, D. McKenna, C. Dooley, E. Sweeney, C. Keane and C. O'Morain (1987) 'Campylobacter pylori and recurrence of duodenal ulcers: a 12-month follow-up study'. *Lancet* 2(8568):1109–11.

Collins, Francis S. (1999) 'Shattuck lecture: medical and societal consequences of the Human Genome Project'. *New England Journal of Medicine* 341:28–37.

Collins, Francis S. and Victor A. McKusick (2001) 'Implications of the Human Genome Project for medical science'. *Journal of the American Medical Association* 285:540–4.

Collins, Harry (2014) *Are We All Scientific Experts Now?* Cambridge: Polity Press.

Connor, Steve (2010) 'Ten years ago today, it was revealed that the human genome had been decoded. A medical revolution beckoned. So what happened next?' *Independent*, 26 June. Online at www.independent.co.uk/news/science/ten-years-ago-today-it-was-revealed-that-the-human-genome-had-been-decoded-a-medical-revolution-2011016.html

Contopoulos-Ioannidis, Despina G., Evangelina Ntzani and John Ioannidis (2003) 'Translation of highly promising basic science research into clinical applications'. *American Journal of Medicine* 114(6):477–84.

Convergence Revolution (2016) *Convergence: The Future of Health*. Online at www.convergencerevolution.net/2016-report

Cotton, P. B., P. R. Salmon, L. H. Blumgart, R. J. Burwood, G. T. Davies, B. W. Lawrie, J. W. Pierce and A. E. Read (1972) 'Cannulation of papilla of Vater via fiber-duodenoscope: assessment of retrograde cholangiopancreatography in 60 patients'. *Lancet* i:53–8.

Cotton, Peter B. (2010) *The Tunnel at the End of the Light: My*

Endoscopic Journey in Six Decades. Marston Gate: Amazon. co.uk Ltd.

Crawford, Matthew B. (2008) 'The limits of neuro-talk'. *New Atlantis*, Winter: 65–78. Online at www.thenewatlantis.com/publications/the-limits-of-neuro-talk

Crimmins, Eileen M. and Hiram Beltrán-Sánchez (2010) 'Mortality and morbidity trends: is there compression of morbidity?' *Journal of Gerontology: Social Sciences* 66B:75–86.

Crofton, John (2006) 'The MRC randomized trial of streptomycin and its legacy: a view from the clinical front line'. *Journal of the Royal Society of Medicine* 99:531–4.

Cronin, A.J. (1937) *The Citadel*. London: Gollancz.

Crook, Amanda (2010) 'Stars buy cancer drugs for Tony'. *Manchester Evening News*, 16 April. Online at www.manchester-eveningnews.co.uk/news/health/stars-buy-cancer-drug-for-tony-997790

Dalrymple, Theodore (2017) 'David Sellu, a surgeon wrongly jailed'. *Spectator Health*, 24 May. Online at https://health.spectator.co.uk/david-sellu-a-surgeon-wrongly-jailed

Danbury, Chris (2017) 'Meeting in the middle: mediation in the medical setting'. *Commentary* (Royal College of Physicians), 16–17 October.

Dancer, S.J. and B.I. Duerden (2014) 'Changes to clinician attire have done more harm than good'. *Journal of the Royal College of Physicians of Edinburgh* 44:293–8.

Darzi, Ara, Harry Quilter-Pinner and Tom Kibasi (2018) *The Lord Darzi Review of Health and Care: Interim Report.*

London: Institute for Public Policy Research. Online at www.ippr.org/files/2018-05/lord-darzi-review-interim-report.pdf

Davies, Andrew (2011) *A. J. Cronin: The Man Who Created Dr Finlay*. Richmond, Surrey: Alma.

Davis, William (2011) *Wheat Belly*. Emmaus, PA: Rodale Inc.

Devine, Oliver, Andrew Harborne, Joshua Kearsley and Ashley Vardon (2016) 'Hold my hand while you misdiagnose me'. *The Clinical Teacher* 13:388–92.

Dicke, W. K. (1950) *Coeliac Disease: Investigation of the Harmful Effects of Certain Types of Cereal on Patients Suffering from Coeliac Disease*. Doctoral Thesis, University of Utrecht.

Dicke, W., H. Weijers and J. van de Kamer (1953) Coeliac disease II: the presence in wheat of a factor having a deleterious effect in cases of coeliac disease'. *Acta Paediatrica Scandinavica* 42:34–42.

Dobson, Roger (2007) 'UK health department criticised for secret deal'. *British Medical Journal* 334:281.

Doll, Richard and A. Bradford Hill (1950) 'Smoking and carcinoma of the lung'. *British Medical Journal* 4682:739–48.

—(1954) 'The mortality of doctors in relation to their smoking habits'. *British Medical Journal* 4877:1451–5.

Donnelly, Laura (2017) '"Game changing" immunotherapy drug denied to AA Gill gets the go ahead'. *Telegraph*, 20 September. Online at www.telegraph.co.uk/news/2017/09/20/game-changing-immunotherapy-drug-denied-aa-gill-gets-go-ahead

Douglas, Colin (1977) *The Greatest Breakthrough since Lunchtime*. Edinburgh: Canongate.

Down, Peter (2013) *A History of Luminal Gastroenterology in Britain.* Weymouth: Watery Books.

Downie, Robin (2016) 'Medical humanities: some uses and problems'. *Journal of the Royal College of Physicians of Edinburgh* 46(4):288–94.

—(2017) 'Patients and consumers'. *Journal of the Royal College of Physicians of Edinburgh* 47:261–5.

Downie, Robin and Fiona Randal (2008) 'Choice and responsibility in the NHS'. *Clinical Medicine* 8:182–5.

Drescher, Jack (2015) 'Out of DSM: depathologizing homosexuality'. *Behavioral Sciences* 5:565–75.

Dr Foster Intelligence (2015) *Uses and Abuses of Performance Data in Healthcare.* Online at www.drfoster.com/updates/recent-publications/uses-and-abuses-of-performance-data-in-health-care

Dubos, René (1959) *Mirage of Health: Utopias, Progress, and Biological Change.* New York: Anchor Books.

Dworkin, Ronald (2000) 'The cultural revolution in health care'. *National Affairs.* Online at www.nationalaffairs.com/public_interest/detail/the-cultural-revolution-in-health-care

Echt, Debra S., Philip R. Liebson, L. Brent Mitchell, Robert W. Peters *et al.* (1991) 'Mortality and morbidity in patients receiving encainide, flecainide, or placebo: the cardiac arrhythmia suppression trial'. *New England Journal of Medicine* 324:781–8.

Edwards, Jim (2010) 'PatientsLikeMe is more villain than victim in patient data "scraping" scandal'. *CBS News*, 19 October. Online at www.cbsnews.com/news/patientslikeme-is-more-villain-than-victim-in-patient-data-scraping-scandal

El-Gingihy, Youssef (2015) *How to Dismantle the NHS in 10 Easy Steps*. Winchester: Zero Books.

Elliot, Chris (2015) 'The problem with the figures on deaths at Stafford Hospital'. *Guardian*, 1 November. Online at www.theguardian.com/commentisfree/2015/nov/01/the-problem-with-the-figures-on-deaths-at-stafford-hospital

Epstein, David and Prorepublica (2017) 'When evidence says no, but doctors say yes'. *The Atlantic*, 22 February. Online at www.theatlantic.com/health/archive/2017/02/when-evidence-says-no-but-doctors-say-yes/517368

Feinstein, Alvan R. (1987) 'The intellectual crisis in clinical science: medaled models and muddled mettle'. *Perspectives in Biology and Medicine* 30:215–30.

—(1995) 'Meta-analysis: statistical alchemy for the 21st century'. *Journal of Clinical Epidemiology* 48:71–9.

—(1996) 'Twentieth century paradigms that threaten both scientific and humane medicine in the twenty-first century'. *Journal of Clinical Epidemiology* 49:615–17.

Feinstein, A. R. and R. I. Horowitz (1997) 'Problems in the "evidence" of "evidence-based medicine"'. *American Journal of Medicine* 103:529–35.

Ferenstein, Gregory (2014) 'Larry Page's wish to make all health data public has big benefits – and big risks'. *Telecrunch*, 19 March. Online at https://techcrunch.com/2014/03/19/larry-

pages-wish-to-make-all-health-data-public-has-big-bene-
fits-and-big-risks/?guccounter=1

Fiennes, Caroline (2016) 'Where your donations to medical
research really go'. *Financial Times*, 28 September. Online at
www.ft.com/content/0d351302-840f-11e6-8897-2359a58ac7a5

Fojo, T., S. Mailankody and A. Lo (2014) 'Unintended consequences of expensive cancer therapeutics: the pursuit of
marginal indications and a me-too mentality that stifles
innovation and creativity: the John Conley Lecture'. *JAMA
Otolaryngology – Head & Neck Surgery* 140:1225–36.

Francis, Robert (2010) *Independent Inquiry Report into Mid-
Staffordshire NHS Foundation Trust*. Online at http://web-
archive.nationalarchives.gov.uk/20130104234315/http://www.
dh.gov.uk/en/Publicationsandstatistics/Publications/Publi-
cationsPolicyAndGuidance/DH_113018

—(2013) *The Mid Staffordshire NHS Foundation Trust Public
Inquiry*. Online at http://webarchive.nationalarchives.gov.
uk/20150407084003/http://www.midstaffspublicinquiry.com

Freedman, David H. (2010) 'Lies, damned lies, and medical
science'. *The Atlantic*, November. Online at https://www.the-
atlantic.com/magazine/archive/2010/11/lies-damned-lies-
and-medical-science/308269

Fries, James F. (1980) 'Aging, natural death, and the compression
of morbidity'. *New England Journal of Medicine* 303:1369–70.

Gill, A.A. (2016) 'More life with your kids, more life with your
friends, more life spent on earth – but only if you pay'. *Sunday Times Magazine*, 11 December.

Gisler, Monika, Didier Sornette and Ryan Woodard (2010) 'Innovation as a social bubble: the example of the Human Genome Project'. *Research Policy* 40:1412–25.

Glasziou, Paul, Amanda Burls and Ruth Gilbert (2008) 'Evidence based medicine and the medical curriculum'. *British Medical Journal* 337:a1253.

GlaxoSmithKline (2016) 'GSK establishes global Immunology Network to collaborate with leading academic research scientists'. Online at https://ie.gsk.com/ie/media/press-releases/2016/gsk-establishes-global-immunology-network-to-collaborate-with-leading-academic-research-scientists

Goldacre, Ben (2014) 'Care.data is in chaos. It breaks my heart'. *Guardian*, 28 February. Online at www.theguardian.com/commentisfree/2014/feb/28/care-data-is-in-chaos

The Goodenough Committee (1944) 'The training of doctors'. *British Medical Journal* 2(4359):121–3.

Goodhart, C. A. E. (1975) 'Problems of monetary management: the UK experience'. In *Papers in Monetary Economics Vol. 1.* Reserve Bank of Australia.

Gray, John (2004) 'An illusion with a future'. *Dedalus* 133(3):10–17.

Greenwood, Major (1931) 'The work of the London School of Hygiene and Tropical Medicine'. *Journal of the Royal Society of Arts* 79:538–48.

Hall, Robert (1986) 'Arthur Hedley Clarence Visick FRCS 1897–1949'. *Annals of the Royal College of Surgeons of England* 68(3):147.

Hall, Stephen S. (2010) 'Revolution postponed'. *Scientific Amer-*

ican, October. Online at https://www.nature.com/scientific-american/journal/v303/n4/full/scientificamerican1010-60.html

Handy, Charles (1994) *The Empty Raincoat: Making Sense of the Future*. London: Hutchinson.

Harari, Yuval Noah (2016) *Homo Deus: A Brief History of Tomorrow*. London: Harvill Secker.

Harbison, Joe (2016) 'Stroke patients are no less deserving than cancer patients'. *Irish Times*, 14 June. Online at www.irishtimes.com/opinion/stroke-patients-are-no-less-deserving-than-cancer-patients-1.2683121

Hardwick, Christopher (1939) 'Prognosis in coeliac disease: a review of seventy-three cases'. *Archives of Disease in Childhood*. Online at www.ncbi.nlm.nih.gov/pmc/articles/PMC1975636

Hart, Julian Tudor (1971) 'The inverse care law'. *Lancet* 1:405–12.

Hawkes, Nigel (2009) 'Patient coding and the ratings game'. *British Medical Journal* 240:c2153.

—(2013) 'How the message from mortality figures was missed at Mid Staffs'. *British Medical Journal* 346:f562.

Hayes, Robert H. and William J. Abernethy (1980) 'Managing our way to economic decline'. *Harvard Business Review*. Online at https://hbr.org/2007/07/managing-our-way-to-economic-decline

Healthcare Commission (2009) *Investigation into Mid-Staffordshire NHS Foundation Trust*. Online at www.nhshistory.net/midstaffs.pdf

Heath, Iona (2006) 'Combating disease mongering: daunting but nonetheless essential'. *PLoS Medicine* 3:e146.

Hedley Visick, Arthur (1948) 'Measured radical gastrectomy: review of 505 operations for peptic ulcer'. *Lancet* i:505–10.

Hernandez, Daniela (2013) 'Selling your most personal item: you'. *Wired.com*. Online at www.wired.com/2013/03/miinome-genetic-marketplace

Herper, Matthew (2017) 'Craig Venter mapped the genome. Now he's trying to decode death'. *Forbes*, 28 February. Online at https://www.forbes.com/sites/matthewherper/2017/02/21/can-craig-venter-cheat-death/#5a07d5911645

Highfield, Roger (2016) 'What's wrong with Craig Venter?' *New Republic*, 2 February. Online at https://newrepublic.com/article/128977/whats-wrong-craig-venter

Hill, Austin Bradford (1985) 'Personal view'. *British Medical Journal* 290:1074.

Hogan, Helen, Rebecca Zipfel, Jenny Neuberger, Andrew Hutchings, Ara Darzi and Nick Black (2015) 'Avoidability of hospital deaths and association with hospital-wide mortality ratios: retrospective case record review and regression analysis'. *British Medical Journal* 351:h3239.

Hogan, Michael (2014) 'The celebrity ice-bucket challenge leaves me cold'. *Daily Telegraph*, 20 August. Online at www.telegraph.co.uk/men/the-filter/11045083/Celebrity-ice-bucket-challenge-why-it-leaves-me-cold.html

Holtzman, Neil A. and Theresa M. Marteau (2000) 'Will genetics revolutionize medicine?' *New England Journal of Medicine* 343:141–4.

Hooker, Claire and Estelle Noonan (2011) 'Medical humanities as expressive of Western culture'. *Medical Humanities* 37: 79–84.

Hopkins, Harold and Narinder Sing Kapany (1954) 'A flexible fibrescope, using static scanning'. *Nature* 173:39–40.

Horton, Richard (2004) 'Why is Ian Kennedy's Healthcare Commission damaging NHS care?' *Lancet* 364:401–2.

—(2015) 'What is medicine's 5 sigma?' *Lancet* 385:1380.

—(2018) 'Offline: "A sea of suffering"'. *Lancet* 391:1465.

Hospice UK (2016) 'Hospice care in the UK 2016'. Online at www. hospiceuk.org/docs/default-source/What-We-Offer/pub-lications-documents-and-files/hospice-care-in-the-uk-2016. pdf?sfvrsn=0

Howick, Jeremy (2011) *The Philosophy of Evidence-Based Medicine*. London: BMJ Books.

Illich, Ivan (1975) *Medical Nemesis – The Expropriation of Health*. London: Calder & Boyars.

Ioannidis, John P. A. (2005) 'Why most published research findings are false'. *PLoS Medicine* 8:e124.

—(2016) 'Evidence-based medicine has been hijacked: a report to David Sackett'. *Journal of Clinical Epidemiology* 73:82–6.

Ioannidis, John P. A., Michael E. Stuart, Shannon Brownlee, Sheri A. Strite (2017) 'How to survive the medical misinformation mess'. *European Journal of Clinical Investigation* 47:795–802.

Jamison, Leslie (2014) *The Empathy Exams: Essays*. Minneapolis: Graywolf Press.

Jansen, Jesse, Vasi Naganathan, Stacy M. Carter, Andrew J. McLachlan, Brooke Nickel and Les Irwig (2016) 'Too much medicine in older people? Deprescribing through shared decision making'. *British Medical Journal* 353:i2893.

Jarman, Brian, Simon Gault, Bernadette Alves, Amy Hider, Susan Dolan, Adrian Cook, Brian Hurwitz and Lisa I. Iezzoni (1999) 'Explaining differences in English hospital death rates using routinely collected data'. *British Medical Journal* 318:1515–20.

Jarrett, Christian (2013) 'A calm look at the most hyped concept in neuroscience: mirror neurons'. *Wired.com.* Online at www.wired.com/2013/12/a-calm-look-at-the-most-hyped-concept-in-neuroscience-mirror-neurons

Jewkes, John (1966) 'A great public issue'. *British Medical Journal* 2:1315–16.

Jokanovic, N., E.C. Tan, M.J. Dooley, C.M. Kirkpatrick and J.S. Bell (2015) 'Prevalence and factors associated with polypharmacy in long-term care facilities: a systematic review'. *Journal of the American Medical Directors Association* 16:535. e1–12.

Kahneman, Daniel (2011) *Thinking, Fast and Slow.* New York: Farrar, Straus and Giroux.

Karlsberg Schaffer, Sarah, Peter West, Adrian Towse, Christopher Henshall, Jorge Mestro-Fernándiz, Robert Masterson and Alastair Fische (2017) 'Assessing the value of new antibiotics: additional elements of value for health technology assessment decisions'. Office of Health Economics. Online at www.ohe.org/system/files/private/publications/OHE%20AIM%20Assessing%20The%20Value%20of%20New%20Antibiotics%20May%202017.pdf

Kelm, Zak, James Womer, Jennifer K. Walter and Chris Feudtner (2014) 'Interventions to cultivate physician empathy: a systematic review'. *BMC Medical Education* 14:219.

Keogh, Bruce (2013) *Review into the Quality of Care and Treatment Provided by 14 Hospital Trusts in England: Overview Report*. Online at www.nhs.uk/NHSEngland/bruce-keogh-review/Documents/outcomes/keogh-review-final-report.pdf

Kevles, Daniel J. (1998) *The Baltimore Case: A Trial of Politics, Science, and Character*. New York: WW Norton.

Kilner, J.M. and R.N. Lemon (2013) 'What we currently know about mirror neurons'. *Current Biology* 23:R1057–62.

Knaul, Felicia Marie, Paul E. Farmer, Eric L. Krakauer, Liliana de Lima *et al.* (2017) 'Alleviating the access abyss in palliative care and pain relief – an imperative of universal coverage: the *Lancet* Commission report'. *Lancet* 391:1391–1454.

Kozubek, Jim (2017) 'The trouble with Big Science'. *Los Angeles Review of Books*, 25 November. Online at https://lareviewofbooks.org/article/trouble-big-science

Krigel, Anna and Benjamin Lebwohl (2016) 'Nonceliac gluten sensitivity'. *Advances in Nutrition* 7:1105–10.

Kroft, Steve (2014) 'The data brokers: selling your personal information'. *CBS News*, 9 March. Online at www.cbsnews.com/news/data-brokers-selling-personal-information-60-minutes

Krugman, Paul (2009) 'Why markets can't cure health care'. *New York Times*, 25 July. Online at https://krugman.blogs.nytimes.com/2009/07/25/why-markets-cant-cure-healthcare

Latham, Jonathan (2011) 'The failure of the genome'. *Guardian*, 17 April. Online at www.theguardian.com/commentisfree/2011/apr/17/human-genome-genetics-twin-studies

Lazarsfeld, Paul Felix and Robert King Merton (1957) 'Mass communication, popular taste and organized social action'. In *Mass Culture: The Popular Arts in America*. Ed. Bernard Rosenberg and David Manning White. New York: Free Press.

Lebwohl, Benjamin, Yin Cao, Geng Zong *et al.* (2017) 'Long term gluten consumption in adults without celiac disease and risk of coronary heart disease: prospective cohort study'. *British Medical Journal* 357:j1892.

Lederle, F. A., D. Zylla, R. MacDonald and T. J. Wilt (2011) 'Venous thromboembolism prophylaxis in hospitalized medical patients and those with stroke: a background review for an American College of Physicians Clinical Practice Guideline'. *Annals of Internal Medicine* 155:602–15.

Legge, Thomas (1934) *Industrial Maladies*. Oxford: Oxford University Press.

Levinovitz, Alan (2015) *The Gluten Lie (And Other Myths about What You Eat)*. New York: Regan Arts.

Lichetta, Mirko and Michael Stelmach (2016) *Fiscal Sustainability Analytical Paper: Fiscal Sustainability and Public Spending on Health*. Office for Budget Responsibility. Online at http://obr.uk/docs/dlm_uploads/Health-FSAP.pdf

Lilford, Richard and Peter Provost (2010) 'Using hospital mortality rates to judge hospital performance: a bad idea that just won't go away'. *British Medical Journal* 340:c2016.

LIPID [The Long-Term Intervention with Pravastatin in Ischemic Heart Disease Study Group] (1998) 'Prevention of cardiovascular events and death with Pravastatin in patients with coronary heart disease and a broad range of initial cholesterol levels'. *New England Journal of Medicine* 339: 1349–57.

Lown, Bernard (1996) *The Lost Art of Healing: Practicing Compassion in Medicine.* Boston: Houghton Mifflin.

Lupton, Deborah (2013) 'The digitally-engaged patient: self-monitoring and self-care in the digital health era'. *Social Theory and Health* 11:256–70.

Lyttleton, R. A. (1979) 'The gold effect'. In *Lying Truths: A Critical Study of Current Beliefs and Conventions.* Ed. R. Duncan and M. Weston-Smith. Elmsford, NY: Pergamon Press.

McCormick, James (1996) 'Medical hubris and the public health: the ethical dimension'. *Journal of Clinical Epidemiology* 49:619–21.

McDonnell, Anthony (2017) 'Providing Orkambi to CF sufferers will cost lives'. *Irish Times*, 20 April. Online at www.irishtimes.com/opinion/providing-orkambi-to-cf-sufferers-will-cost-lives-1.3051756

McKeown, Thomas (1988) *The Origins of Human Disease.* Oxford: Basil Blackwell.

—(1979) *The Role of Medicine: Dream, Mirage, or Nemesis?* Princeton: Princeton University Press.

McNamara, Robert S. (1995) *In Retrospect: The Tragedy and Lessons of Vietnam.* New York: Time Books.

Macnaughton, Jane (2009) 'The dangerous practice of empathy'. *Lancet* 373:1940–1.

Makary, Martin A. and Michael Daniel (2016) 'Medical error: the third leading cause of death in the US'. *British Medical Journal* 353:i2139.

Mandrola, John (2014) 'Good doctoring is not rocket science: it is also not digital'. Online at https://medcitynews.com/2014/06/good-doctoring-rocket-science-also-digital

Manolio, Teri A., Francis S. Collins, Nancy J. Cox *et al.* (2009) 'Finding the missing heritability of complex diseases'. *Nature* 461:747–53.

Marcus, Gary (2012) 'Neuroscience fiction'. *The New Yorker*, 30 November. Online at www.newyorker.com/news/news-desk/neuroscience-fiction

Marshall, B.J., C.S. Goodwin, J.R. Warren, R. Murray, E.D. Blincow, S.J. Blackbourn, M. Phillips, T.E. Waters and C.R. Sanderson (1988) 'Prospective double-blind trial of duodenal ulcer relapse after eradication of Campylobacter pylori'. *Lancet* 2(8626–8627):1437–42.

Meades, Jonathan (2017) 'In the loop'. *Times Literary Supplement*, 18 October. Online at www.the-tls.co.uk/articles/public/arts-and-art-meades

Medawar, Peter (1980) 'In defence of doctors'. *New York Review of Books*, 15 May.

Meskó, Bertalan (2017) *The Guide to the Future of Medicine.* Self-published under Webicina Kft.

Minkel, J.R. (2008) 'Scientists know better than you – even

when they're wrong'. *Scientific American*, 9 May. Online at www.scientificamerican.com/article/scientists-know-better-than-you

Mohammed, M. A., R. Lilford, G. Rudge, R. Holder and A. Stevens (2013) 'The findings of the Mid-Staffordshire Inquiry do not uphold the use of hospital standardized mortality ratios as a screening test for "bad" hospitals'. *Quarterly Journal of Medicine* 106:849–54.

Monaghan, Gabrielle (2016) 'Rory Staunton: the boy who died from a gym class scrape'. *Irish Independent*, 13 October. Online at www.independent.ie/life/rory-staunton-the-boy-who-died-from-a-gym-class-scrape-35125789.html

Morgan, G., R. Ward and M. Barton (2004) 'The contribution of cytotoxic chemotherapy to 5-year survival in adult malignancies'. *Clinical Oncology* 16:549–60.

Motzer, Robert J., Thomas E. Hutson, Piotr Tomczak *et al.* (2009) 'Overall survival and updated results for Sunitinib compared with Interferon Alfa in patients with metastatic renal cell carcinoma'. *Journal of Clinical Oncology* 27:3584–90.

Moynihan, Ray, Iona Heath and David Henry (2002) 'Selling sickness: the pharmaceutical industry and disease mongering'. *British Medical Journal* 324:886–90.

National Institute of Clinical Excellence (2017) 'Nivolumab for previous treated squamous non-small-cell lung cancer'. Online at www.nice.org.uk/guidance/ta483

Naughton, John (2018) 'How Theranos used the media to create the emperor's new startup'. *Guardian*, 3 June. Online at www.

theguardian.com/commentisfree/2018/jun/03/theranos-eliz-abeth-holmes-media-emperors-new-startup

Obituary. (2009) 'Robert McNamara'. *The Economist*, 9 July. Online at www.economist.com/obituary/2009/07/09/robert-mcnamara

O'Donnell, Michael (1971) 'Decorated municipal gothic'. *World Medicine* 7:101.

O'Mahony, Denis and Paul Francis Gallagher (2008) 'Inappro-priate prescribing in the older population: need for new cri-teria'. *Age and Ageing* 37:138–41.

O'Mahony, Seamus (2012) 'AJ Cronin and *The Citadel*: did a work of fiction contribute to the foundation of the NHS?' *Journal of the Royal College of Physicians of Edinburgh* 42: 172–8.

—(2013) 'Against Narrative Medicine'. *Perspectives in Biology and Medicine* 56:611–19.

—(2014) 'How scientific inquiry works'. *Dublin Review of Books*, April, Issue 54. Online at www.drb.ie/essays/how-scientific-inquiry-works

—(2014) 'John Bradshaw (1918–1989): putting doctors on trial'. *Irish Journal of Medical Science* 184:559–63.

—(2015) 'In praise of Richard Asher (1912–1969)'. *Perspectives in Biology and Medicine* 57:512–23.

—(2015) 'Truculent priest'. *Dublin Review of Books*, November, Issue 72. Online at www.drb.ie/essays/truculent-priest

—(2016) *The Way We Die Now*. London: Head of Zeus.

—(2016) '*Medical Nemesis* 40 years on: the enduring legacy of

Ivan Illich'. *Journal of the Royal College of Physicians of Edinburgh* 46:134–9.

—(2017) 'Medicine and the McNamara fallacy'. *Journal of the Royal College of Physicians of Edinburgh* 47:281–7.

—(2017) 'A postmodern disease'. *Dublin Review of Books*, February, Issue 86. Online at www.drb.ie/essays/a-postmodern-disease

—(2017) 'Compassion, empathy, flapdoodle'. *Dublin Review of Books*, September, Issue 92. Online at www.drb.ie/essays/compassion-empathy-flapdoodle

—(2018) 'Some thoughts on compassion inspired by Sir Thomas Legge'. *Journal of the Royal College of Physicians of Edinburgh* 48:69–70.

O'Neill, Des (2017) 'Empathy is for the long haul: think about it'. *Irish Times*, 23 May. Online at www.irishtimes.com/life-and-style/health-family/empathy-is-for-the-long-haul-think-about-it-1.3086419

O'Neill, Onora (2002) *A Question of Trust*. Cambridge: Cambridge University Trust.

Ortega y Gasset, José (1944) *Mission of the University* (translated by Howard Lee Nostrand). Princeton: Princeton University Press.

Pappworth, Maurice (1967) *Human Guinea Pigs: Experimentation on Man*. London: Routledge.

Paris, Joel (2013) *Fads and Fallacies in Psychiatry*. London: RCPsych Publications.

Perlmutter, David (with Kristin Loberg) (2014) *Grain Brain*. London: Hodder & Stoughton.

Pettypiece, Shannon and Jordan Robertson (2014) 'Hospitals are mining patients' credit card data to predict who will get sick'. *Bloomberg.com*. Online at www.bloomberg.com/news/articles/2014-07-03/hospitals-are-mining-patients-credit-card-data-to-predict-who-will-get-sick

Platt, John R. (1964) 'Strong inference'. *Science* 146:347–53.

Pollock, Allyson (2002) 'Comment: We work in teams but are blamed as individuals'. *GMC News* 10:2.

Poole, Steven (2012) 'Your brain on neuroscience: the rise of popular neurobollocks'. *New Statesman*, 6 September. Online at www.newstatesman.com/culture/books/2012/09/your-brain-pseudoscience-rise-popular-neurobollocks

Porter, Roy (1997) *The Greatest Benefit to Mankind: A Medical History of Humanity from Antiquity to the Present.* London: HarperCollins.

Powell, J. Enoch (1966) *A New Look at Medicine and Politics.* London: Pitman Medical.

—(1976) *Medicine and Politics: 1975 and After.* London: Pitman Medical.

Prasad, Vinay, Andrae Vandross, Caitlin Toomey *et al.* (2013) 'A decade of reversal: an analysis of 146 contradicted medical practices'. *Mayo Clinic Proceedings* 88:790–8.

Pye, David (2016) 'If we know so much about disease, where are all the cures?' *The Conversation*. Online at https://theconversation.com/if-we-know-so-much-about-disease-where-are-all-the-cures-58955

Ramachandran, V.S. (2011) *The Tell-Tale Brain: A Neuroscientist's*

Quest for What Makes Us Human. New York: WW Norton & Co.

Ramesh, Randeep (2013) 'Mid-Staffs A&E closure: Sir Brian Jarman career profile'. *Guardian*, 28 July. Online at www.theguardian.com/society/2013/jul/28/mid-staffs-closure-brian-jarman-profile

Rees, Martin (2003) *Our Final Century*. London: William Heinemann.

Rennie, Drummond (1986) 'Guarding the guardians: a conference on editorial peer review'. *Journal of the American Medical Association* 256(17):2391–2.

Reuters (2016) 'Cancer Moonshot program is "close to gigantic progress", Joe Biden says'. *Guardian*, 17 October. Online at www.theguardian.com/us-news/2016/oct/17/joe-biden-cancer-moonshot-program-update

Rhee, Chanu, Shruti Gohil and Michael Klompas (2014) 'Regulatory mandates for sepsis care: reasons for caution'. *New England Journal of Medicine* 370:1673–6.

Rich, Joseph (2018) 'Doctors, revolt!' *New York Times*, 24 February. Online at www.nytimes.com/2018/02/24/opinion/sunday/doctors-revolt-bernard-lown.html

Richards, Sarah Elizabeth (2018) 'Can genetic counselors keep up with 23andMe?' *The Atlantic*, 22 May. Online at www.theatlantic.com/health/archive/2018/05/can-genetic-counselors-keep-up-with-23andme/560837

Richmond, Caroline (2002) 'Dame Sheila Sherlock'. *British Medical Journal* 324:174.

Riess, Helen (2010) 'Empathy in medicine: a neurobiological perspective'. *Journal of the American Medical Association* 304:1604–5.

Riess, Helen, John M. Kelley, Robert W. Bailey, Emily J. Dunn and Margot Phillips (2012) 'Empathy training for resident physicians: a randomized controlled trial of a neuroscience-informed curriculum'. *Journal of General Internal Medicine* 27:1280–6.

Roberts, Sam (2017) 'Uwe Reinhardt, 80, dies; a listened-to voice on health care policy'. *New York Times*, 15 November. Online at www.nytimes.com/2017/11/15/obituaries/uwe-reinhardt-a-listened-to-voice-on-health-care-policy-dies-at-80.html

Robinson, Gerry (2013) 'Yes we can fix the NHS'. *Daily Telegraph*, 17 February. Online at www.telegraph.co.uk/news/health/news/9876178/Yes-we-can-fix-the-NHS-says-Gerry-Robinson.html

Rory Staunton Foundation (2013) 'Rory's Regulations'. Online at https://rorystauntonfoundationforsepsis.org/rorys-regulations-full-legal-document

Rosenweig, Phil (2010) 'Robert S. McNamara and the evolution of modern management'. *Harvard Business Review*. Online at https://hbr.org/2010/12/robert-s-mcnamara-and-the-evolution-of-modern-management

Ruane, Thomas J. (2000) 'Correspondence: is academic medicine for sale?' *New England Journal of Medicine* 343:508–10.

Rumbold, John and Sarah Seaton (2016) 'Mid-Staffs: disaster by numbers (or How to create a drama out of a statistic)?' *Journal of Medical Law and Ethics* 4:57–70.

Sackett, David L., R. Brian Haynes and Peter Tugwell (1985) *Clinical Epidemiology: A Basic Science for Clinical Medicine.* Boston: Little, Brown & Co.

Sackett, David L. and Andrew D. Oxman (2003) 'HARLOT plc: an amalgamation of the world's two oldest professions'. *British Medical Journal* 327:1442–5.

Sackett, David L., William M. C. Rosenberg, J. A. Muir Gray, R. Brian Haynes and W. Scott Richardson (1996) 'Evidence based medicine: what it is and what it isn't'. *British Medical Journal* 312:71–2.

Salinas, Joel (2017) *Mirror Touch: Notes from a Doctor Who Can Feel Your Pain.* New York: HarperCollins.

Samet, Jonathan M. and Frank E. Speizer (2006) 'Sir Richard Doll, 1912–2005'. *American Journal of Epidemiology* 164(1):95–100.

Sapone, Anna, Julio C. Bai, Carolina Ciacci *et al.* (2012) 'Spectrum of gluten-related disorders: consensus on new nomenclature and classification'. *BMC Medicine* 10:13. Online at https://bmcmedicine.biomedcentral.com/track/pdf/10.1186/1741-7015-10-13

Saunders, Cicely (2006) *Selected Writings 1958–2004.* Oxford: Oxford University Press.

Schoenfeld, Jonathan D. and John P. A. Ioannidis (2013) 'Is everything we eat associated with cancer? A systematic cookbook review'. *American Journal of Clinical Nutrition* 97:127–34.

Scottish Conservative and Unionist Party Manifesto (2016) 'A world-class health care system for your loved ones'. Online at www.scottishconservatives.com/wordpress/wp-content/uploads/2016/04/Scottish-Conservative-Manifesto_2016-DIGITAL-SINGLE-PAGES.pdf

Scottish Conservatives (2017) 'New figures reveal years of SNP failure on waiting times'. Online at www.scottishconserva-tives.com/2017/02/new-figures-reveal-years-of-snp-failure-on-waiting-times

Seife, Charles (2013) '23andMe is terrifying, but not for the reasons the FDA thinks'. *Scientific American*, 29 November. Online at www.scientificamerican.com/article/23andme-is-terrifying-but-not-for-the-reasons-the-fda-thinks

Seldon, Joanna (2017) *The Whistleblower: The Life of Maurice Pappworth*. Buckingham: University of Buckingham Press.

Seymour, Christopher W., Foster Gesten, Hallie C. Prescott *et al.* (2017) 'Time to treatment and mortality during mandated emergency care for sepsis'. *New England Journal of Medicine* 376:2235–44.

Shah, Hriday M. and Kevin C. Chung (2009) 'Archie Cochrane and his vision for evidence-based medicine'. *Plastic & Recon-structive Surgery* 124(3):982–8.

Shaw, George Bernard (1909) *The Doctor's Dilemma: Preface on Doctors*. Online at https://ebooks.adelaide.edu.au/s/shaw/george_bernard/doctors-dilemma/preface.html

Shepherd, James, Stuart M. Cobbe, Ian Ford, Christopher G. Isles, A. Ross Lorimer, Peter W. McFarlane, James H. McKillop and Christopher J. Packard (1995) 'Prevention of coronary heart disease with Pravastatin in men with hypercholesterolaemia'. *New England Journal of Medicine* 333:1301–8.

Singer, Natasha (2010) 'When patients meet online, are there side effects?' *New York Times*, 29 May. Online at www.nytimes.com/2010/05/30/business/30stream.html

Skrabanek, Petr (1986) 'Demarcation of the absurd'. *Lancet* 1(8487):960–1.

—(1988) 'The physician's responsibility to the patient'. *Lancet* 331:1155–7.

—(1990) 'Nonsensus consensus'. *Lancet* 335(8703):1446–7.

—(1994) *The Death of Humane Medicine and the Rise of Coercive Healthism*. London: The Social Affairs Unit.

—(2000) *False Premises, False Promises: Selected Writings of Petr Skrabanek*. Glasgow: Tarragon Press.

Skrabanek, Petr and James McCormick (1989) *Follies and Fallacies in Medicine*. Glasgow: Tarragon Press.

Smaldino, Paul E. and Richard McElreath (2016) 'The natural selection of bad science'. *Royal Society Open Science* 3(9): 160384. Online at http://rsos.royalsocietypublishing.org/content/3/9/160384

Smith, Richard (2001) 'Why are doctors so unhappy?' *British Medical Journal* 322:1073.

—(2003) 'Limits to medicine. Medical nemesis: the expropriation of health'. *Journal of Epidemiology and Community Health* 57:928.

—(2011) *The Trouble with Medical Journals*. London: The Royal Society of Medicine Press.

—(2016) 'Epidemiology: big problems and an identity crisis'. *BMJ blogs*, 10 October. Online at https://blogs.bmj.com/bmj/2017/03/09/richard-smith-can-we-look-forward-to-a-healthier-future/

—(2017) 'Can we look forward to a healthier future?' *BMJ blogs*, 9 March. Online at https://blogs.bmj.com/bmj/2017/03/09/richard-smith-can-we-look-forward-to-a-healthier-future

—(2017) 'Schopenhauer, the economist, and cancer'. *BMJ blogs*, 22 September. Online at https://blogs.bmj.com/bmj/2017/09/22/richard-smith-schopenhauer-the-economist-and-cancer

—(2018) 'A Big Brother future for science publishing?' *BMJ blogs*, 10 January. Online at https://blogs.bmj.com/bmj/2018/01/10/richard-smith-a-big-brother-future-for-science-publishing

Smith, Richard and David Pencheon (2017) 'Disavowal: the great excuser that may destroy us'. *BMJ blogs*, 4 September. Online at https://blogs.bmj.com/bmj/2017/09/04/richard-smith-and-david-pencheon-disavowal-the-great-excuser-that-may-destroy-us

Smith, Richard and Drummond Rennie (2014) 'Evidence-based medicine: an oral history'. *British Medical Journal* 348:g371.

Socialist Health Association (1969) *Report on Ely Hospital*. Online at www.sochealth.co.uk/national-health-service/democracy-involvement-and-accountability-in-health/complaints-regulation-and-enquries/report-of-the-committee-of-inquiry-into-allegations-of-ill-treatment-of-patients-and-other-irregularities-at-the-ely-hospital-cardiff-1969

Sokal, Alan D. (1996) 'Transgressing the Boundaries: Towards a Transformative Hermeneutics of Quantum Gravity'. *Social Text* 46/47:217–52.

Spiegelhalter, David (2013) 'Have there been 13,000 needless deaths at 14 NHS trusts?' *British Medical Journal* 347:f4893.

Sullivan, Richard and the *Lancet* Oncology Commission (2011) 'Delivering affordable cancer care in high-income countries'. *Lancet Oncology* 12:933–80.

Sweeney, Kieran, Domhnall MacAuley and Denis Pereira Gray (1998) 'Personal significance: the third dimension'. *Lancet* 10:134–6.

Swinford, Steven, Laura Donnelly and Patrick Sawer (2013) 'Labour's "denial machine" over hospital death rates'. *Daily Telegraph*, 14 July. Online at www.telegraph.co.uk/news/health/heal-our-hospitals/10178552/Labours-denial-machine-over-hospital-death-rates.html

Tainter, Joseph A. (1988) *The Collapse of Complex Societies.* Cambridge: Cambridge University Press.

Tait, Ian (1982) 'Dubos' Mirage of Health'. *Journal of the Royal College of General Practitioners* 32:248.

Tallis, Raymond (2004) *Hippocratic Oaths: Medicine and Its Discontents.* London: Atlantic Books.

Taylor, Paul (2013) 'Rigging the death rate'. *London Review of Books*, 11 April. Online at https://www.lrb.co.uk/v35/n07/paul-taylor/rigging-the-death-rate

—(2014) 'Standardized mortality ratios'. *International Journal of Epidemiology* 42:1882–90. Online at https://academic.oup.com/ije/article/42/6/1882/743648

Tedeschi, Bob (2017) 'Doctors have resisted guidelines to treat sepsis. New study suggests those guidelines save lives'. Online at https://rorystauntonfoundationforsepsis.org/7771/stat news-doctors-resisted-guidelines-treat-sepsis-doctors-resisted-guidelines-treat-sepsis-new-study-suggests-guidelines-save-lives

Tennant, Jon (2018) 'Scholarly publishing is broken: here's how to fix it'. *Aeon*. Online at https://aeon.co/ideas/scholarly-publishing-is-broken-heres-how-to-fix-it

Tett, Gillian (2018) 'Digital medicine: bad for our health?' *Financial Times*, 2 February. Online at www.ft.com/content/3ed1cc6c-0612-11e8-9650-9c0ad2d7c5b5

Thomas, Kas (2017) 'The never-ending war on cancer'. Online at https://bigthink.com/devil-in-the-data/the-never-ending-war-on-cancer

Thomas, Lewis (1983) *The Youngest Science: Notes of a Medicine Watcher.* New York: Viking Press.

Thompson, Sylvia (2018) 'Patient organisations shouldn't have to march on the streets to get access to medicines'. *Irish Times*, 21 June. Online at www.irishtimes.com/special-reports/patient-healthcare/patient-organisations-shouldn-t-have-to-march-on-the-streets-to-get-access-to-medicines-1.3529125

Topol, Eric (2015) *The Patient Will See You Now.* New York: Basic Books.

United European Gastroenterology Research (2014) 'Healthcare in Europe: scenarios and implications for digestive and liver diseases'. Online at https://d3lifz0r4hvny1.cloudfront.net/

fileadmin/user_upload/documents/press/ueg_week_2014_-_
press_releases/futurescenarios/uk_futurescenarios_press-
release.pdf

Vacher, Louise (2015) 'Understanding the FreeFrom consumer'.
Online at www.fdin.org.uk/wp-content/uploads/2015/10/
Understanding-The-Freefrom-Consumer-Louise-Vacher-
YouGov.pdf

Van Berge-Henegouwen, G. P. and C. J. J. Mulder (1993) 'Pioneer
in the gluten-free diet: Willem-Karel Dicke 1905–1962, over
50 years of gluten free diet'. *Gut* 34:1473–5.

Van de Kamer, J. H., H. A. Weijers and W. K. Dicke (1953)
'Coeliac disease. IV: an investigation into the injurious con-
stituents of wheat in connection with their action on patients
with coeliac disease'. *Acta Paediatrica* 42:223–31.

Van Epps, Heather L. (2006) 'René Dubos: unearthing antibiotics'. *Journal of Experimental Medicine* 203(2):259.

Varmus, Harold (2010) 'Ten years on: the human genome and
medicine'. *New England Journal of Medicine* 362:2028–9.

Ventola, C. Lee (2015) 'The antibiotic resistance crisis, part 1:
causes and threats'. *Pharmacy & Therapeutics* 40:277–83.

Verghese, Abraham (2009) 'In praise of the physical examination'. *British Medical Journal* 339:b5448.

—(2010) 'Beyond measure: teaching clinical skills'. *Journal of
Graduate Medical Education* 2(1):1–3.

Vokes, E. E., N. Ready, E. Felip *et al.* (2018) Nivolumab versus
docetaxel in previously treated advanced non-small-cell lung
cancer (CheckMate 017 and CheckMate 057): 3-year update

and outcomes in patients with liver metastases'. *Annals of Oncology* 29:959–65.

Vrecko, Scott (2010) 'Neuroscience, power and culture: an introduction'. *History of the Human Sciences* 23(1):1–10.

Wade, Nicholas (2010) 'A decade later, genetic map yields few new cures'. *New York Times*, 12 June. Online at www.nytimes.com/2010/06/13/health/research/13genome.html

Weatherall, D. J. (1994) 'The inhumanity of medicine'. *British Medical Journal* 309:1671–2.

—(1996) *Science and the Quiet Art: The Role of Medical Research in Health Care*. London: WW Norton.

Weinberg, Alvin M. (1967) *Reflections on Big Science*. Cambridge, MA: MIT Press.

Weinberg, Robert A. (2014) 'Coming full circle – from endless complexity to simplicity and back again'. *Cell* 157:267–71.

Weiner, Tim (2009) 'Robert S. McNamara, architect of a futile war, dies at 93'. *New York Times*, 7 July. Online at www.nytimes.com/2009/07/07/us/07mcnamara.html

Wellcome Witnesses to Twentieth Century Medicine (2000) *Peptic Ulcer: Rise and Fall*. London: Wellcome Foundation. Online at www.histmodbiomed.org/sites/default/files/44836.pdf

Westaby, Stephen (2017) 'The shaming of heart surgeons: how politics brought a proud profession low'. *Spectator Health*, 16 February. Online at https://health.spectator.co.uk/the-shaming-of-heart-surgeons-how-politics-brought-a-proud-profession-low/

White House: Office of the Press Secretary (2000) 'Remarks made by the President, Prime Minister Tony Blair of England (via satellite), Dr Francis Collins, Director of the National Human Genome Research Institute, and Dr. Craig Venter, President and Chief Scientific Officer, Celera Genomics Corporation, on the completion of the first survey of the Entire Human Genome Project'. Online at www.genome.gov/10001356/june-2000-white-house-event

Wijesuriya, Jeeves (2017) 'Why the case of Dr Hadiza Bawa-Garba makes doctors so nervous'. *New Statesman*, 2 February. Online at www.newstatesman.com/politics/health/2018/02/why-case-dr-hadiza-bawa-garba-makes-doctors-so-nervous

Williams, Roger, R. Y. Calne and I. D. Ansell *et al.* (1969) 'Liver transplantation in man, III: studies of liver function, histology and immunosuppressive therapy'. *British Medical Journal* 3:12–19.

Wilson, Duncan (2011) 'Who guards the guardians? Ian Kennedy, bioethics and the 'Ideology of Accountability' in British medicine'. *Social History of Medicine* 25:193–211.

Wise, Peter H. (2016) 'Cancer drugs, survival, and ethics'. *British Medical Journal* 355:i5792.

Wright, Ronald (2005) *A Short History of Progress*. Edinburgh: Canongate.

Yankelovich, Daniel (1972) *Corporate Priorities: A Continuing Study of the New Demands of Business*. Stanford, CT: Yankelovich Inc.

INDEX